Neuropsychological Treatment
of Dyslexia

Neuropsychological Treatment of Dyslexia

DIRK J. BAKKER

Translated by Ginny Spyer

New York   Oxford
OXFORD UNIVERSITY PRESS
1990

Oxford University Press   9-22-93

Oxford   New York   Toronto
Delhi   Bombay   Calcutta   Madras   Karachi
Petaling Jaya   Singapore   Hong Kong   Tokyo
Nairobi   Dar es Salaam   Cape Town
Melbourne   Auckland

and associated companies in
Berlin   Ibadan

Originally published in The Netherlands as
*Zijdelings: Neuropsychologische Methoden
ter Behandeling van Dyslexieën,*
copyright © 1987 by Dirk J. Bakker
and Swets & Zeitlinger B.V.

Library of Congress Cataloging-in-Publication Data
Bakker, Dirk J.
[Zijdelings. English]
Neuropsychological treatment of dyslexia
by Dirk J. Bakker : translated by Ginny Spyer.
p.   cm.   Translation of : Zijdelings.
Includes bibliographical references.
ISBN 0-19-506132-2
1. Dyslexia—Treatment.   2. Clinical neuropsychology.
I. Title. [DNLM: 1. Brain—physiopathology.
2. Dyslexia—rehabilitation.   3. Neuropsychology.
WL 340 B168z]   RC394.W6B3513   1990   616.85'5306—dc20
DNLM/DLC   for Library of Congress   89-22946   CIP

9 8 7 6 5 4 3 2 1

Printed in the United States of America
on acid-free paper

Foreword

Interest in the remediation of developmental dyslexia is as old as the discovery of the condition itself. The physicians who first described the disorder in the early years of the century assumed that cerebral abnormality—specifically, maldevelopment of the inferior posterior parietal region of the left hemisphere—was responsible for the occurrence of "congenital wordblindness." However, even though they postulated a structural basis for the disability, they were not at all despairing about the prospects of treating it. On the contrary, they urged that special training procedures outside the regular classroom be utilized with dyslexic children, and they expressed confidence that the disability could be alleviated if not entirely eliminated. James Hinshelwood, the leading investigator in this early period, recommended specific methods designed to strengthen sight–sound associations such as the use of block letters for spelling words. Some clinicians advocated employment of the "look and say" method, instead of the then prevailing phonetic approach to the teaching of reading. Still others suggested that reading-disabled children be taught to write with the left hand in order to facilitate utilization of the homologous region of the right hemisphere in the mediation of reading.

Through the decades, numerous methods of remediation, based upon one or another theory of the nature and cause of specific reading disability, have been used with dyslexic children. The underlying conceptions have been diverse in character, ranging from the anatomophysiological (as in the early concept of congenital wordblindness) to the purely psychological. The remedial methods derived from these conceptions have been equally diverse, ranging from pharmacologic intervention to behavior modification based on Skinnerian principles.

Professor Dirk Bakker has been an active investigator in the field of developmental dyslexia for many years, his first publication on the topic dating back to 1965. His research has been marked by two salient characteristics: First, it has been pursued within the framework of contemporary developments in clinical neuropsychology, particularly those concerned with the role of cerebral hemispheric asymmetry in the mediation of cognitive processes, a field to which he himself has made notable contributions. Second, as head of a research department devoted to the remediation of learning disabilities, his ultimate goal has been to develop more effective procedures to help learning-disabled children overcome their handicaps.

Professor Bakker's monograph reflects both of these characteristics. His research indicates that although reading is clearly a bihemispheric process, it is one in which each hemisphere makes a distinctive contribution at successive stages as a young child learns to read. A significant number of (but not all) dyslexic children show one or another type of imbalance as they face the task of learning to read. Proceeding from these empirical findings, he and his students have devised instructional methods designed to correct an observed imbalance. Reading-disabled children taught by these methods have shown gratifying progress.

Professor Bakker not only has presented an account of some highly original neuropsychological studies of the reading process, but also has subjected the educational implications of his findings to empirical testing. Possessing both theoretical and practical significance, his work will command the attention of neuropsychologists, reading specialists, and teachers.

Arthur Benton

Preface
to the English Edition

> There is no more merit in having
> read a thousand books than in
> having ploughed a thousand fields.
> WILLIAM SOMERSET MAUGHAM

For many years the research carried out in the Child Neuropsychology Department of the Pedological Institute in Amsterdam has focused on the causes and treatment of dyslexia. The fruits of this endeavor have usually been communicated in English and typically in technical jargon. In Holland, the need gradually arose to summarize the results of this research in an orderly and comprehensive fashion so that interested professionals—neuropsychologists, psychologists, neurologists, psychiatrists, educators, and teachers in special education—could work with it therapeutically and educationally. Accordingly, the Dutch version of this book was written. As some people felt that an English translation would be worthwhile, the present version came into being.

This book documents only a small part of all the research being conducted in the complex field of dyslexia; however, it should be noted that in comparison with other areas of research, relatively few resources have been devoted to the scientific study of dyslexia. This is remarkable, because dyslexia afflicts millions of children and adults throughout the world and, like other learning disabilities, can lead to feelings of self-doubt, guilt, resentment, rage, despair, reproach, a general inability to cope, and sometimes even suicidal tendencies—in short, to emotional instability, depression, and social isolation. These disconcerting words were used by Dr. Thomas E. Bryant, director of the U.S. President's Commission on Mental Health, in his report to President Carter (*Bulletin of the Orton Society,* 1978, *28:* 8–14). In a recent large-scale study of the sequelae of learning disability in children of primary school age, Dr. Otfried Spreen found considerable social and economic implications for later life: "Not only do these youngsters suffer through a miserable and usually shortened school career, live a discouraging social life, full of disappointments and failures, they also have fewer chances for adequate employment and advanced training" (*Learning-Disabled Children Growing Up;* Lisse: Swets & Zeitlinger, 1987, p. 133). Certainly a problem of this scope should not be addressed by only a few researchers, having inadequate resources and funding.

This book was translated by Ginny Spyer M.A., one of my associates, who is well acquainted with the subject matter. I owe her and Rosalind Corman, copy editor, many thanks for their conscientious and resourceful work. I am grateful also to Dr. Robin Morris (Atlanta) and Dr. Harry Van der Vlugt (Tilburg) who read the text and proposed some improvements. Of course, they are not responsible for any possible inaccuracies that may have remained in the text. Jeffrey House (Oxford University Press) and Klaus Plasterk (Swets & Zeitlinger), who first opened up discussion on the production of an English version, are thanked for their initiative. I am honored that Dr. Arthur Benton (Iowa City), my scientific mentor, was willing to write a Foreword.

Neuropsychological Treatment of Dyslexia differs from the original Dutch version in some respects. A new section (5.5) on recent studies was added, a few other sections were expanded, and still others were abbreviated. Words used as treatment material, as displayed in some figures, are either translated or presented in Dutch. In the latter case, the reader should have no difficulty in understanding the treatment being discussed. In the interest of readability, few references are cited in the text. This book is not intended as a primary source in itself but rather a summary or compilation of works listed in the Bibliography. One may find Chapters 7, 8, and 9 to be somewhat impersonal and technical. However, the didactic approach used in these chapters is necessary to elucidate the steps to be performed in the course of the various therapies.

It is hoped that the methodical approach employed will help one avoid any misconceptions.

Dyslexia is a handicap from which many suffer; it must be eradicated. As long as this goal has not yet been reached, suffering of dyslexics would be eased if our societies realized that there is more between heaven and earth than reading and writing alone: there are many fields that need to be ploughed. I hope that this book will inspire researchers and clinicians to take on the challenge, as well as funding agencies to expand their level of commitment to research on dyslexia.

Amsterdam   *D.J.B*

Contents

Neuropsychological Treatment
of Dyslexia

1

A Set of Brains

1.1. Left–Right Inside

In the Dutch language, one invariably speaks of brain*s*—that is, in the plural. There is something to be said for this. Within the skull there are two half-spheres—a left and a right cerebral hemisphere. In Figure 1, the brain is viewed from above; thus both hemispheres can be discerned easily. A deep groove runs longitudinally over the brain. The floor of this groove is formed by the corpus callosum, one of the most important connections between the left and the right hemispheres. The outer layer of the brain is called the *cortex* (or bark). The cortex is extremely wrinkled and convoluted, so that it has a very large surface area.

Billions of nerve cells constitute the basic units of the brain. Figure 2 depicts a *nerve cell* (*neuron*), which consists of a cell body (soma) and (usually) many branches (axon and dendrites). Nerve cells conduct *electric impulses* and generally transmit them to one another. These electric currents, although extremely weak, can be made visible by means of an *electroencephalogram* (*EEG*).

The brain is the "seat of all behavior." Perceiving—that is, seeing, hearing, feeling, smelling, tasting, as well as remembering, learning, speaking, reading, calculating, and moving—are possible only with the assistance of our brain. Each type of behavior can be traced to one particular part of the brain more than to another. To a certain degree, the brain can be viewed as an assembly of specialists (*not* soloists). The sections in the rear of the cortex (the occipital lobes) are specialized in sight; the sides (the temporal lobes), in audition; the top sections (the parietal lobes), in touch.

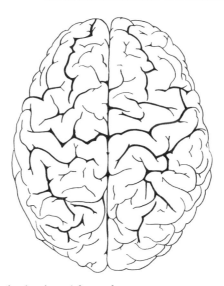

FIGURE 1. The brain viewed from above.

The intermediate sections and those situated toward the front of the cortex (the frontal lobes) are concerned primarily with other, extremely complex *behaviors* (functions).

In terms of specialized functions, there is an important difference between the left and right halves of the brain. For the great majority of people, the left hemisphere is specialized (dominant) for language, and the right hemisphere for the perception of form and direction. Damage to the left side of the brain is usually ac-

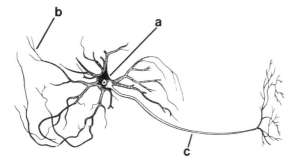

FIGURE 2. A nerve cell: (a) the cell body; (b) dendrites; (c) axon.

companied by speech and language disabilities; an injury to the right usually leaves these functions intact. When one reads, one is engaged in language. Thus, reading activates the left hemisphere. But, in the course of reading, one also perceives letter *forms,* which are ordered in a left-to-right *direction.* Therefore, reading is a function also of the right hemisphere.

More nerve tissue is found *beneath* the cortex than *within* the cortex. This lower–upper dimension of the brain, as essential as it may be, is of minor import for the present discussion.

1.2. Left–Right Outside

There is a left and a right cerebral hemisphere. There is also a left and a right hand, foot, eye, and ear. One can easily add to this list. Left and right are thus present not only inside the brain (*centrally*), but also outside it (*peripherally*).

Within the periphery, an important distinction (for the present discussion) can be made between the left and right *visual fields*. These visual "half-fields" can be formed by holding a pencil upright in one's hand and stretching one's arm so that the point of the pencil is at eye level. If one were now to look at the point of the pencil (the *fixation point*), then one will have formed, to the left of this point, the left visual field, and to the right of it, the right visual field. It should be evident that the left and right visual fields do *not* correspond to the left and right eye, respectively.

1.3. Outside Left–Inside Right and Outside Right–Inside Left

The left and right outside and inside of the brain are closely connected. Generally speaking, one can say that left in the periphery is connected predominantly to the right cerebral hemisphere, and vice versa.

We shall illustrate the cross-relationship between outside and inside by means of the visual half-fields. Suppose that one is looking (and continues to look) at point X in Figure 3. The regions to the left and right of this point are the visual half-fields. Suppose,

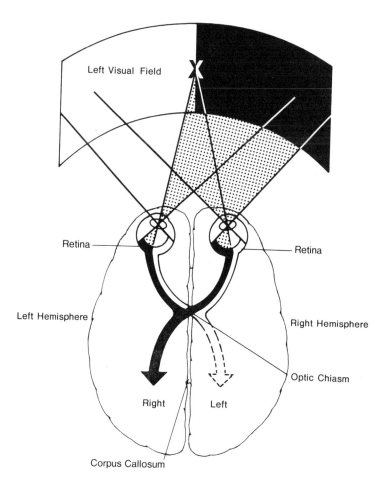

FIGURE 3. Crossed relationship between left visual field and right
hemisphere (the "white" tract), and right visual field and left hemisphere (the "black" tract), respectively. Retina: the light-sensitive
surface at the back of the eye. Optic chiasm: a junction in the brain
where visual information crosses over to the opposite sides of the
brain. (After S. C. Levine, Hemispheric specialization and functional
plasticity during development. In M. Frank (Ed.), *A Child's Brain*.
New York: Haworth Press, 1984.)

6

furthermore, that one is shown the word "book" in the left visual field. In this case, "book" is received by the right hemisphere. Another way of saying this is that "book" is *projected* to the right hemisphere and, more specifically, to the posterior (occipital) region of the right hemisphere (*visual cortex*). Whatever one sees in the left visual field activates primarily the nerve cells in the visual cortex of the right hemisphere. Understandably, objects viewed in the right visual field activate primarily the visual cortex of the left hemisphere.

The hands display a similar outside–inside relationship. When one handles a plastic letter with the fingers of the left hand, it is primarily the somatosensory cortex of the parietal region of the right hemisphere that is activated. In the same manner, the left somatosensory cortex is activated when one touches an object with the right hand.

With regard to audition, the outside–inside relationship is somewhat more complex. The left ear projects to the right as well as to the left hemisphere (temporal region), although predominantly to the right auditory cortex. The right ear projects predominantly, though not exclusively, to the auditory cortex of the left hemisphere.

2

The Brain and
Learning to Read

2.1. Words in a Sentence

We have already seen that when words are presented to the left
and right visual fields, they are projected to the visual cortex of
the right and left hemispheres, respectively. As was also mentioned previously, the left and right visual fields are those areas to
the left and right of the fixation point at which one is looking.

When one is reading a book, as the reader is doing now, one's
eyes "jump" from left to right across the sentence, using "jumps"
(*eye movements*) from fixation point to fixation point. These fixations last only a fraction of a second. The more experienced one is
in reading, the fewer fixations one displays per sentence; that is,
one makes bigger "jumps." Suppose that at a certain point one
fixates in the middle of a word in a sentence, in the word "book"—
that is, *bo* x *ok* (where x is the fixation point)—for example. The
letters *bo* (and whatever precedes that) are thus perceived in the
left visual field, and *ok* (and whatever follows that) in the right
visual field. Thus, *bo* is projected to the right hemisphere, and *ok*
to the left. One nevertheless reads "book," because all regions of
the brain cooperate with one another.

We now know that words that are presented within either the
left or the right visual field are projected to the visual cortex of
the right and left hemispheres, respectively. When one is reading
ordinary text, words are presented in both visual fields simultaneously, and are thus projected simultaneously to the visual cortex
of both the right and left hemispheres.

What happens *after* the right and/or left visual cortices have been activated? This activity definitely does not remain restricted to the visual cortex. When a written (printed) word has to be perceived, designated, comprehended, and articulated, activity of the entire brain is called for. Even so, one part of the brain will display more activity than another.

2.2. Hemispheres and Learning to Read

The left hemisphere is more involved in common, everyday reading than is the right hemisphere. This rule of thumb holds true for most adult readers. When adults read, the balance of brain activity is tipped toward the left; the right hemisphere *participates,* but to a lesser degree. By common reading, we mean activities such as the reading of a book, magazine, or newspaper.

Once in a while, one is confronted with uncommon reading material. In advertising brochures, for example, complex letter-types are sometimes used. The typeface reproduced in Figure 4 is an extreme example.

Considerable effort is required to unravel this uncommon script. We call it *perceptually complex,* in contrast to common script, which we call *perceptually simple.* There is evidence that the reading of uncommon script activates the right hemisphere to a larger extent than does the reading of common script. The relatively large participation of the right hemisphere in the reading of uncommon script is probably due to the perceptual complexity (and/or "novelty") of the material. The right hemisphere is known to be activated when one needs to discriminate forms and directions (such as left–right, under–above).

At a certain point in time, a child begins learning to read. The child is presented with script. For adults, these letters and words are familiar and perceptually simple. Is this true also for the child? There are a great many letters and other symbols. These letters are sometimes difficult to distinguish from one another. Many mistakes are possible: A "d" could be viewed as a "b," "p," or "q." Turn an "m" or "n" upside down, and something akin to a "w," "v," or "u" results. But this is not all. The word "name" could be read as "mean," "mane," "amen," or something else if the child doesn't read the letters from left to right. On the other

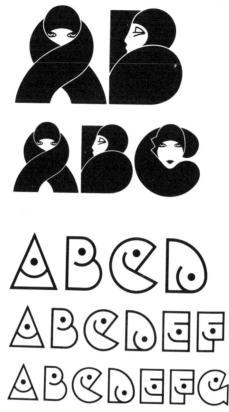

FIGURE 4. Uncommon lettertypes. (After *Graphic book*. Le Perray-en-Yuelines, France: Mecanorma Industries.)

hand, "name," "Name," "NAME," *"N A M E,"* and even "nAMe" are all the same words, whether they are printed in black, white, green, red, or blue. The left-to-right sequence of the words in a sentence also determines the meaning of that sentence. The sentence "he is here" has a different meaning from "is he here" or "here he is."

Letters, words, and sentences are peculiar, perceptually complex phenomena for the child at the outset of the learning-to-read process. Thus, one must assume that *initial reading* is controlled more by the right than by the left hemisphere. But as the child grows older and passes from one grade to the next, the strange letters and words gradually become more familiar. The perceptual complexity of the script starts to wane. The child learns to read without having to perceive every letter or every word. These letters and words are "filled in" on the basis of the *language experience* that the child has acquired. The reading, which initially was slow, has gained speed. In short, initial reading becomes advanced, adult reading. This form of reading is controlled predominantly by the left hemisphere.

In initial reading, the balance of brain activity favors the right hemisphere, whereas advanced reading favors the left hemisphere. Thus, there is a moment in the learning-to-read process at which the balance in the brain tips from right to left.

The above discussion has referred to *brain activity* during reading. This activity can be measured with the aid of EEG techniques. We recorded *event-related potentials* (*ERPs*) during the reading of words, in children who consecutively passed through the last year of kindergarten and the first three grades of elementary school. Thus, the sequence went from no reading, to initial reading, and then to advanced reading. Did the balance of brain activity tip from right to left? Before answering this question, we should first characterize these ERPs.

2.3. Brain Activity and Reading

Being largely made up of nerve cells, the brain continuously produces electricity. This electricity can be recorded on the outside of the skull by means of little metal plates—electrodes—which are glued to the scalp with conductive paste. The electric currents that are detected are extremely weak—on the order of millionths of a volt (microvolts)! With the use of amplifiers, these signals can nevertheless be made manifest on a rolling sheet of paper, on which writing pins reproduce the electric activity of the brain in the form of waves (EEG).

The brain produces electricity continuously, not only during waking states, but also during sleep. The characteristics of the wave pattern—the height of the waves and their number per second—depends upon many factors, such as the age of the

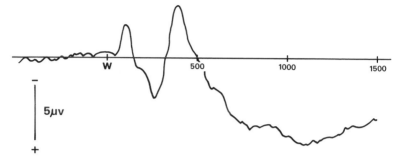

FIGURE 5. Electric response of the brain to the presentation of words. (After Bakker & Vinke, 1985; ref. 2.)

person and the activities he or she is performing during EEG registration. A special kind of EEG, the *ERP,* or event-related potential, registers electric potentials (P), which emerge as a specific reaction (R) to an event (E). An event can be a variety of things: The presentation of a word flashed on a screen, for example, induces a *word-related potential* (*WRP*). The electric potential is thus the response of the brain to the presentation of the word. This kind of response is depicted in Figure 5. The W in the figure is the moment at which the word is presented. After the presentation of W, a "hill and valley" pattern emerges for a short period of time (in the figure, 1500 milliseconds (ms) = 1.5 seconds), which reflects the response of the brain. The "hills and valleys" have a maximum height and depth, called *amplitudes.* The moment at which the positive and negative slopes reach their greatest height/depth, counting from W, is called the *latency period.* In Figure 5, the first peak has an amplitude of approximately 3 microvolts (mV) and a latency of 100 ms. On account of this latency and the fact that at this point the electric potential is *negative* (a "hill"), this peak is denoted as *N100.* Now it should not be difficult for one to deduce what is designated as *P250* (P stands for positive) and *N500,* in Figure 5. The N500 is followed by a long, drawn-out positive wave (the *slow positive-wave*). The amplitudes and latencies in Figure 5 exemplify the mean electric responses to a large series of word presentations.

ERPs can be recorded basically anywhere on the skull. In

practice, however, one usually works with certain, often symmetrical, locations on the left and right sides of the skull. Thus, P3 and T3 (i.e., uneven numbers) are sites on the skull above the parietal and temporal regions, respectively, of the left hemisphere, whereas P4 and T4 (i.e., even numbers) are sites situated above these same regions of the right hemisphere. It is not uncommon that the amplitude and latency of a wave from the left and right sides of the skull differ. In this case, there is *asymmetry* in the activity of the cerebral hemispheres.

2.4. Progressing from Initial to Advanced Reading

A previously mentioned study involved children who successively passed through the last year of kindergarten and the first three grades of elementary school; thus they developed from nonreaders, to beginning readers, and then to advanced readers. The question posed by the investigators concerned the balance of hemispheric activity; did it tip from right to left in the course of this progression?

Because the children could not read at the first encounter, they were taught a number of simple words. Once the children were acquainted with them, these words were flashed (many times in succession) on a screen. Electrodes were attached to the left and right sides of the skull (T3 and T4; P3 and P4) in these children so that word-related potentials (WRPs) could be recorded. The whole procedure was repeated after one, two, and three years. Additional evaluations were carried out as well; for example, reading and spelling tests were also administered.

The results of the study demonstrated that the *asymmetry* (the left–right difference *between* the hemispheres) of some of the WRP amplitudes changed with the progression of the learning-to-read process. Certain amplitudes were larger in the right hemisphere at the toddler age, and larger in the left at a more advanced age.

Reading and spelling abilities, which, as mentioned above, were also studied, proved to be related to the WRP amplitudes in the right hemisphere at an early age and to those in the left hemisphere at more advanced ages. These results indicate that the balance of hemispheric activity does indeed tip from right to left with

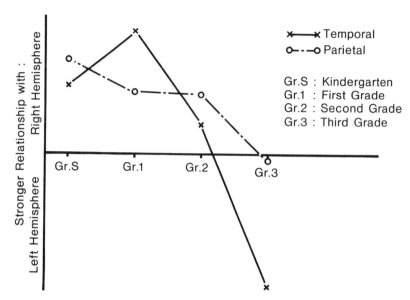

FIGURE 6. Development of the relationship between reading/language ability and hemispheric activity, as measured at temporal and parietal sites of the brain. (After Licht, Bakker, Kok, & Bouma, 1988; ref. 72.)

the progression of the learning-to-read process (Fig. 6). The switch appears to take place at the end of the first or the beginning of the second grade.

These results to a large extent correspond with those obtained from visual half-field investigations. The relation between visual half-fields and the cerebral hemispheres was discussed in Chapter 1, Section 1.3. The right visual field projects to the left hemisphere, the left field to the right hemisphere. One can flash words in both fields and request that these words be read. In adults, one often finds that words presented to the right are read more accurately and/or more swiftly than those presented to the left. On the basis of such results, it has been concluded that words are more effectively processed in the left hemisphere (i.e., the *right* visual field is superior; thus, the *left* hemisphere is superior).

The results of a number of visual half-field studies revealed a remarkable difference between younger and older elementary school children. Older children, like adults, produced superior reading performance when the reading material was presented in the right visual field. In contrast, young children (up to approximately 8 years of age) read best in the left visual field. Initial reading, in contrast to advanced reading, appears to be a function more of the right than the left hemisphere. The results of some visual half-field studies, as well, suggest that the "switch in hemisphere" takes place at 7 to 8 years of age.

3

Dyslexias

3.1. Reading Disabilities: "Betting on the Wrong Horse"

Suppose that a child wants to learn to ride horseback. There are two horses, L and R, that are quite different in character and have quite diverse capabilities. Horse L is swift and experienced with the rules of trotting. The other horse, R, is slow but a keen observer. The child has never been on a horse before. With which horse shall it begin? R is the preferable horse. The pupil will gradually become acquainted with the peculiarities of the horse. R is composed, and a good observer as well: He will trot and look out for hurdles and obstacles. This saddle is a safe one, and very few riding mistakes will be made.

Our pupil now wants to become a jockey, an elegant and swift horseback rider. Horse R was a good start, but our pupil cannot win a prize with it in a derby. This goal is attainable only with the swift and skilled horse, L. If the pupil wants to become a jockey, he or she will, after some time, have to switch to L, on penalty of a stagnation in the learning-to-ride process. To start with horse R is fine, but to continue on it will lead to a "dysjockia" of the type R.

And what if the pupil begins instead with L? This choice will lead to falls, not because of the horse's inexperience, but on account of the rider's. If L takes a hurdle quickly, L's body will contract, and the pupil might be dislodged. Riding will be swift, but mistakes will be made. The pupil will not become a jockey, but is at risk of developing a "dysjockia" of the L type.

One should understand that the letters L and R in our metaphor

16

have been chosen deliberately; L stands for left, and R for right hemisphere. Every comparison falls short, however; no reader "rides" solely the left or solely the right hemisphere. However, the intention of the metaphor should be obvious.

Initial or beginning reading requires a perceptual analysis of the form and direction of letters and words. It is the right hemisphere that most keenly observes and evaluates these hurdles and obstacles. For this reason, initial reading will profit from the mobilization of *right hemispheric strategies.*

But initial reading must eventually become fluent or advanced reading. This phase can be reached only if the horses are switched, only if the "principal seat" of reading shifts from the right to the left hemisphere. If this fails to occur, the reader will become stuck in a slack style of reading, characterized by a perceptual bias. A dyslexia of the P (perceptual) type will develop. *P-dyslexics* appear to remain persistently sensitive to the perceptual characteristics of the text. The letters possess for them an object rather than a symbol character. P-dyslexics are relatively slow although accurate readers. They have a functionally overdeveloped right hemisphere or an underdeveloped left hemisphere (or both) for the processing of reading material.

Whereas some readers begin correctly (using right hemispheric strategies) and wind up wrong (P-dyslexics), others set off to a wrong start: From the very start, they "bet on the fast horse." These young readers make use of predominantly left hemispheric strategies. These strategies are based on "language experience" and are linguistic in nature. These can be effective only when the perceptual features of the text no longer require much attention, which is the case only in an advanced phase of the learning-to-read process. During initial reading, however, these features call for a great deal of attention. Perceptual negligence in this phase therefore leads to many reading errors. A premature mobilization of left hemispheric strategies in reading can lead to a dyslexia of the L type (linguistic). *L-dyslexics* are relatively fast but inaccurate readers. They possess a functionally overdeveloped left or an underdeveloped right hemisphere (or both) for the processing of reading material.

3.2. L- and P-Dyslexia: Characteristics

Dyslexics of the L and P type employ predominantly left and right hemispheric reading strategies, respectively. An obvious question that could be asked is whether the *reading styles* of these types differ. It has already been proposed that L-dyslexics are relatively fast but inaccurate readers, and that P-dyslexics are characterized by a relatively slow but accurate reading style. The results of investigations carried out with a large number of neurological patients with brain damage lend support to this hypothesis. During the execution of tasks related to reading, patients with a damaged right but an intact left hemisphere show a fast but inaccurate mode of action, whereas patients with a damaged left and an intact right hemisphere work fairly accurately, albeit slowly. The combination *fast–inaccurate* appears to characterize left hemispheric activity, whereas the combination *slow–accurate* characterizes that of the right hemisphere. Thus in order to differentiate L- and P-dyslexics, one could ascertain the time required to read a fragment of text (speed) and the number of errors made (accuracy). The L-dyslexics would be the *relatively* fast–inaccurate readers, and the P-dyslexics the *relatively* slow–accurate ones.

To classify L- and P-dyslexia, it would seem, in principle, sufficient to examine the speed and accuracy of reading. Nevertheless, other characteristics of reading style have also been taken into account. If one acknowledges the fact that not all errors are equal, one can discriminate between *substantive* and *time-consuming* errors. Substantive errors include omissions and additions of letters and words, word mutilations, and such—in short, all "real" mistakes. Time-consuming errors are not really errors at all but instead involve words that are initially read in a fragmented (spelling-like) and/or repetitive fashion, but are eventually read correctly. Substantive errors are considered to be characteristic of L-dyslexics (*inaccuracy factor*), whereas time-consuming errors are considered to be characteristic of P-dyslexics because stammering and repetitiveness result in slackness of reading (*time factor*). It thus seems possible to discriminate L- and P-type dyslexia on the basis of speed and accuracy on the one hand, and the type of errors made during reading, on the other hand. We should mention that attempts have been made to detect other type-related characteristics. As a result of these investigations, we can say that L-dyslexics are inclined possibly toward a right-ear advantage, and P-dyslexics toward a left-ear advantage (on dichotic listening tasks). To comprehend the reason for this finding, one should recall that the right and the left ear project predominantly to the left and the right hemisphere, respectively (Chap. 1, Sec. 1.3). Suppose someone is presented with a number of different words in the right and left ear simultaneously, and is requested to repeat the words heard. The result of this kind of *dichotic listening* test is usually that words presented to the right ear are repeated more accurately than those presented to the left ear. A person who produces this result is said to have a right-ear advantage (i.e., a right-ear advantage for spoken language). A right-ear advantage indicates that the left hemisphere is dominant in the processing of spoken language. For certain reasons, one may *not* assume, however, that a left-ear advantage always indicates dominance of the right hemisphere. It is safe to say, nevertheless, that spoken language is processed in the left hemisphere in the case of a right-ear advantage, and (more or less) bilaterally in the case of a left-ear advantage.

How does *ear advantage* relate to reading in general, and more specifically, to the L/P classification? Reading—or, more specifically, reading aloud—is not possible without spoken language. When a dyslexic is inclined to make use predominantly of the left hemisphere in the processing of text, and furthermore displays dominance of the left hemisphere for spoken language, this dyslexic will be all the more inclined to develop left hemispheric strategies in reading. To put it another way, it is certain that he or she will be a dyslexic of the L type. Conversely, a dyslexic with a left-ear advantage, who is already inclined toward activation of the right hemisphere when reading, will inevitably be a dyslexic of the P type.

In summary, we argued that L- and P-dyslexics can be classified on the basis of the dimensions fast + inaccurate versus slow + accurate, substantive errors versus time-consuming errors, and a right- versus a left-ear advantage. If these dimensions have been chosen correctly, then one might expect that they are interrelated—that there is an interrelationship among left-ear advantage, time-consuming errors, and slowness of reading, and among right-ear advantage, substantive errors, and fast reading. At the time of writing, such a relationship has not as yet been researched exhaustively. However, various studies have demonstrated a relationship between a right-ear advantage and substantive errors, and between a left-ear advantage and time-consuming errors.

In addition to the possible interrelationships among these variables, there is the plausible connection between these dimensions and the activity of the cerebral hemispheres during reading. After all, the difference in activity of the left and right hemisphere is the foundation upon which the L/P classification rests. For this reason, if dyslexics, classified as L and P types according to the dimensions enumerated above, differ in the degree in which their cerebral hemispheres are activated during reading, then the classification developed according to these dimensions is reliable. In other words, the question, Is the L/P classification valid?, must be addressed.

3.3. Is the Concept of L- and P-Dyslexia Valid?

On the basis of reading style (speed of reading, nature of the errors) and ear advantage, a great number of children with reading disabilities can be classified as dyslexics of the L and P type. During reading, L-dyslexics and P-dyslexics use predominantly left and right hemispheric strategies, respectively. In other words, when L-dyslexics read, the *balance of brain activity* tips toward the left, whereas when P-dyslexics read, it tips toward the right. As stated previously, brain activity can be measured by means of WRPs—electric potentials produced by the reading of presented words.

In one investigation, L- and P-dyslexics were requested to read words that were flashed in the *central* visual field. WRPs in the temporal and parietal zones of the left and right hemisphere were recorded. The amplitudes of the negative waves (in the temporal zones) proved to be larger in the left than in the right hemisphere in L-dyslexics, whereas this left–right difference was not present in the P-dyslexics.

In another study, L- and P-dyslexics were investigated twice in a similar manner, with an interval of nine months between testing. It was of interest to determine whether, during this period, a type-specific development (i.e., where the development of L-dyslexics differed from that of P-dyslexics) in the use of the cerebral hemispheres occurred during reading. It turned out that in L-dyslexics the electric activity of the left hemisphere had increased after nine months; in other words, they were L types to a greater extent than before. In P-dyslexics, the activity of the right hemisphere had increased; thus they had plunged even more deeply into P-type dyslexia.

In a recent study, L- and P-type dyslexic boys, as well as their biological parents, were administered a number of neuropsychological tests. The original L/P classification was based on type of reading errors made (substantive vs. time-consuming) and the time needed for reading a passage of text (slow vs. fast reading). On the basis of the neuropsychological test results, 82% of the boys and 72% of their fathers could be correctly classified as L or P type.

The results of these and other investigations certainly indicate that the L/P classification is not unfounded. More to the point, existing evidence suggests that the classification is valid.

3.4. How Can L- and P-Dyslexics Be Distinguished?

What is dyslexia? It may seem strange, but this is not an easy question to answer. An airtight definition does not exist. Dyslexia can be defined romantically as a faint star in a star-studded sky. This means that the reading and language achievements of the dyslexic stand in stark contrast to the "firmament" of his or her abilities. He or she exhibits a language deficit in the midst of talents.

For that matter, it is becoming increasingly evident that it is inappropriate to speak of *the* dyslexic. One dyslexic is not the same as another—there are types. The L and P types are examples. The L/P classification is not exhaustive; we have never succeeded in classifying more than 60% of all dyslexics as L or P. There are two possible reasons for our failure to construct an exhaustive classification. In the first place, it is possible that other dyslexias exist, in addition to L and P. Indeed, it is not improbable, in view of the results of research being conducted elsewhere. Moreover, the measuring instruments used in classifying dyslexics may not be entirely accurate. If one were to measure a wall with a piece of rope or with the length of an arm, then the conclusion that the wall is 10 meters long should be taken with a grain of salt; one could easily be a few decimeters off. At the time of writing this book, the same holds true for the L/P classification of dyslexia. With the instruments currently employed to measure dyslexia, it is quite possible, for example, that an L-dyslexic will be overlooked or unjustly classified as such. However, this does not mean that the entire L/P classification is suspect. After all, if this were so, the validation studies (see Sec. 3.3) would not have yielded any useful results. But for the sake of clarity, one should be aware that the classification of L-dyslexics and P-dyslexics still requires some improvements.

To date, the identification of L- and P-type dyslexics has been carried out as follows: Children who, according to their teachers, have marked reading difficulties are given a text to read whose level of difficulty is somewhat higher than their own. Reading errors are classified as *substantive* (real)—for example, omissions, additions, and word mutilations—or as *time-consuming*—for example, fragmentations and repetitions. Furthermore, one *might wish* to administer a dichotic listening test (in which numbers or letters/words can be used) a number of times, in order to ascertain whether the child has a right- or a left-ear advantage (or neither of these). The dichotic listening test should be administered several times because there are indications that the more often the instrument is administered to a child, the more reliable the results become.

After administration of the reading tests, the children are ranked according to the number of errors they have made of each type (substantive and time-consuming). If a child has made more than the average number of substantive errors, in addition to less than the average number of time-consuming errors, then it is assumed that the child is an L-type dyslexic. Those children who score below average on substantive errors and above average on time-consuming errors are considered to be P-type dyslexics. It is as yet uncertain whether it would not perhaps be more appropriate to take into consideration the amount of time necessary for the child to read an excerpt of text instead of the number of time-consuming errors. Needing little time plus making many errors is an indication of L-dyslexia, whereas the combination of much time and few errors indicates P-dyslexia.

One might wonder how to determine, in the context of a daily school routine, whether an individual dyslexic is of the L or P type (or neither). One could determine whether a dyslexic child, in comparison to other dyslexic children, reads very hastily and makes a great many mistakes. Perhaps the opposite is encountered—that is, extreme slowness of reading accompanied by a large number of fragmentations. The former and latter child display characteristics of the L and P type, respectively. Unfortunately, a standardized testing instrument by which one could classify L- and P-dyslexics in a more reliable fashion does not yet exist, but it is currently being worked on in Dutch populations.

4

Neuropsychological
Treatment Methods

4.1. Hemisphere-Specific Stimulation

In reading, dyslexics of the L type get off to a wrong start. From the very beginning, they tackle script predominantly with left hemispheric strategies, whereas right hemispheric strategies are essential in the starting phase of the learning-to-read process. Obviously, a newcomer to the skill of reading should have an eye for the direction and form characteristics of the text.

But in L-type dyslexics, the right hemisphere does not wish to "join in," and now the question is, What can be done to persuade this hemisphere to come along? A logical answer could be to *stimulate* the right hemisphere. This stimulation must be aimed *specifically* toward the right, and as little as possible toward the left hemisphere. Such stimulation can be accomplished by presenting all reading material in the left visual field. This material would then *be projected to*—that is, *received by*—the right hemisphere. Of course, the material—or more correctly, the information—does not remain solely in the right hemisphere. The left hemisphere is needed as well, for complete processing of the text (words, for example). Nevertheless, the "landing site" is the right hemisphere.

The goal of such stimulation is to make the right hemisphere more active in order to effect changes in the strategy (style) of reading: fewer mistakes and slower reading. It is, after all, the right hemisphere that is being stimulated, and the characteristics "slow" and "accurate" characterize this hemisphere.

P-dyslexics set off to a good "reading start" by mobilizing predominantly right hemispheric strategies. But in a later stage of the learning-to-read process, they fail to switch to left hemispheric strategies. Therefore, it might be possible to help P-dyslexics by stimulating the left hemisphere in order to compel greater participation of this hemisphere during reading.

Our expectation is that such stimulation will lead to greater activity in the left hemisphere and thus to a change in reading strategy—specifically, greater speed, but also perhaps some loss in accuracy. Obviously, inaccuracy is undesirable. While inaccuracy possibly might follow from breaking with a wrong strategy, it can perhaps be overcome quickly if appropriate measures are taken.

Direct stimulation of the right hemisphere in L-dyslexics and of the left hemisphere in P-dyslexics is called *hemisphere-specific stimulation (HSS)*. One might anticipate that this kind of stimulation will improve only certain aspects of reading (accuracy, for example), but not all reading skills.

Hemisphere-specific stimulation can take place via the visual half-fields. In principle, the tactile and auditory channels may be addressed as well. In order to stimulate the right hemisphere (in L-dyslexics), one can present the reading material by touch (tactile stimulation) to the fingers of the left hand. One can also address several channels simultaneously—for example, by presenting words in the left/right visual field, asking the subject to read words aloud, and then conducting these articulations to the left/right ear. When making use of the auditory channel, one should bear in mind that the ear does not project exclusively to one hemisphere.

Hemisphere-specific stimulation via the visual channel is not as easy to carry out as one might expect. The difficulty lies in the *control of fixation*. It is important to recall that the visual half-fields exist only if the child stares at a certain point (fixation point). How to control for fixation during presentations in the visual half-fields will be elucidated later on. It is not a simple task, and therefore, easier methods for stimulating the right/left hemisphere have been sought.

4.2. Hemisphere-Alluding Stimulation

Hemisphere-specific stimulation via the visual half-fields is not easy to accomplish. The equipment required is rather costly, and the es-

sential control of fixation requires a certain amount of resourceful-
ness. For this reason, the question was raised, during discussions
held with teachers, as to whether one could stimulate each of the
cerebral hemispheres by using simpler methods—for example, ordinary reading books.

In an earlier section (Chap. 2, Sec. 2.1), we explained that the
words in a sentence that are to be read are "received" by both
hemispheres, and that after these words are "received," the entire
brain is activated. One could, however, attempt to revise the words
in a sentence in such a way that, although still being received by
both hemispheres, they will now make a stronger appeal to the
right or to the left hemisphere during the rest of their processing.
Because of the revision they have undergone, these words are
passed on, as it were, to one of the cerebral hemispheres.

Suppose that in the process of reading a book, the words are being projected to both hemispheres; now suppose that one wants to
alter the process so that a strong appeal is made to the right hemisphere. In other words, one wants the text to *allude* (*alludere:*
Latin for "refer to") to the right hemisphere. In order to achieve
this, one could print the text in an unusual and complicated fashion—for instance, by using various typefaces. In this way, the letter and word forms that are to be processed have become perceptually complex. The right hemisphere is specialized in the analysis
of form and direction; thus the perceptually complex script activates this hemisphere toward greater participation in the reading
process. This is exactly what L-dyslexics need. Training with perceptually laden texts could thus be of therapeutic value for dyslexia of the L type. Figure 7 gives an example of perceptually laden
text.

Now, with respect to P-dyslexics, how should script be altered
in order to allude to the left hemisphere? Can common texts be
revised in such a way that the left hemisphere is activated more
strongly? If the answer is yes, then the presentation of this kind of
reading material should be of some help to P-dyslexics. The left
hemisphere has a number of specialized functions, among them
the analysis of speech sounds and the temporal ordering (ordering
in time) of these sounds. Sound analysis can be accomplished by
rhyming and *temporal ordering,* through placing the letter sounds
of a word in the proper order. Figure 8 is a text fragment in which

LucHtbelℓen

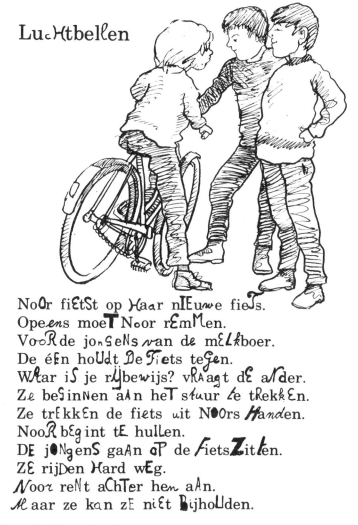

NoOr fiEtSt op Haar nIEuwe fieJs.
Opeens moeT Noor rEmMen.
VooRde jonℊeNs van de mELℛboer.
De éEn hoUdt De Fiets teℊen.
WℛAar iS je rℓjbewijs? vRAaℊt dE aℛder.
Ze beℊinNen aAn het stuur ℓe tRekkEn.
Ze trEkkEn de fiets uit NⲟOrs Handen.
NooR bEℊint tE huLLen.
DE jⲟNℊenS gaAn oT de FietsZitℛen.
ZE rijDen Hard wEg.
Noor reNt aChTer hen aAn.
ℳaar ze kan zE niEt BijhoLLden.

FIGURE 7. Example of perceptually laden text. (After Schrijverscollectief: *De avonturen van Noor en de Kinderen om de Hoek 2*. Baarn: Bekadidact, 1977.)

I read a book   I like to chop wood
I fish with a ....   My coat has a ....

As blind as a mole   The girl is not old
My sock has a .....   The soup is not .....

He sleeps like a log
To bark like a ......

FIGURE 8.   Finding the missing word by using rhyme.

the missing words can be found by means of rhyming to a previous word. Once the word "hook" (Figure 8, first stanza) has
been articulated, one can ask which letter was pronounced *first*
("h"), which *next* ("o"), and so forth (temporal order of the
letters).

It goes without saying that the texts designed for P-dyslexics
should contain the *minimum* number of elements possible that
could allude to the right hemisphere. Uncommon lettertypes,
colors, and illustrations should be avoided. Hemisphere-specific
and hemisphere-alluding stimulation can be combined, for example, by training L-dyslexics with perceptually complex words that
are presented in the left visual field. Other combinations of both
stimulation techniques are not difficult to imagine.

4.3. Is the Brain Pliable?

Heavy rainfall increases the rate of flow of the water in a river. If
the skies clear, then the water in the river will, after a while, re-
gain its initial rate of flow. The current thus reacts to the presence
and absence of rain. Likewise, the brain reacts to stimulation and
to the degree of stimulation.

The question can be raised as to whether the river is still exactly
the same river before and after the heavy rainfall. At first glance,
it appears to be the same, but in reality it is not. If it rains constantly over many seasons, there will be consequences for the riverbed. It will wear away and thereby become deeper. The banks
might cave in, and tributaries might form. In short, the *"struc-*

ture," the "hardware" of the river will eventually change, and with it its *"function";* because the riverbed has become deeper and/or wider, more water will be able to flow through it.

Does the structure, and with it the function, of the brain undergo modifications when it is constantly stimulated richly and unvaryingly by the environment? Evidently so, and the story of the young rats reared in different environments can serve as an illustration. Rats that had been reared in a "dull" cage were compared to peers that had spent the first part of their lives in a sociable cage. A sociable, enriched cage, in contrast to a dull, impoverished cage, has seesaws, ladders, and wheels in various colors, and also many playmates. The brains of the richly stimulated rats were found to differ in appearance from those of rats reared in impoverished cages. In the case of the former, for example, certain areas of the cortex were found to be comparatively thicker, to contain larger nerve cells, with more branchings. Thus, in response to the question posed above, the brain appears to be structurally pliable under the influence of stimulation from the environment.

We had to pose this question because if hemisphere-specific or hemisphere-alluding stimulation proved to have positive effects on reading and spelling, then we could assume that changes in the stimulated hemisphere were responsible for these reading and spelling effects. Thus the concept is that through (sustained) stimulation, the brain or parts of the brain are altered in such a way that reading and spelling ability are favorably influenced (Figure 9).

It is difficult to discover what actually occurs in the human brain

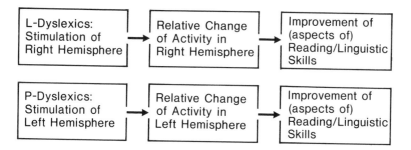

FIGURE 9. Scheme of the effects of stimulation of the hemispheres in L- and P-dyslexics.

as a result of *psychological stimulation,* but by comparing recordings made before and after protracted hemisphere-specific and
-alluding stimulation, it is possible to determine whether the electrophysiological activity of the hemispheres has changed, because
such changes are reflected in the EEG.

Hemisphere-specific and hemisphere-alluding stimulation are
intended not solely to improve reading and spelling abilities of
dyslexics, but are designed also to relate these improvements to
changes in the physiological activity of the stimulated hemispheres.
Since we will be discussing research pertaining to this relationship,
it was necessary to clarify beforehand that the structure and the
function of the cerebral hemispheres can be modified to a certain
degree by specific psychological stimulation.

5
Results of Neuropsychological Treatment

5.1. Control Studies

Let us suppose that a dyslexic child is treated with a new method for three months, and that after this period of time, it is determined that the child reads better than before. May one then conclude that the new treatment has been effective? By no means! The child is three months older, and it could very well be that his or her reading has improved for this reason alone. Another possibility is that the increment in reading is related to the warm, stimulating person carrying out the treatment, or is due to the extra attention the child received. Improvement *after* a treatment is not the same thing as improvement *because* of a treatment.

It is not a simple matter to arrive at a reliable assessment of the efficacy of a therapy. This is possible only if concurrent circumstances that might have played a role during the treatment have been brought under control. How this is done can be clarified with an example, which also serves as an introduction to the remaining chapters, in which the results of hemisphere-specific and -alluding stimulation are discussed.

If one wishes to ascertain, for example, whether right hemispheric stimulation has an effect on the reading ability of L-type dyslexic children, one cannot limit oneself to stimulating these children for a while in order to ascertain what effect this stimulation has had on reading ability. One ought to look at the effects of right-hemispheric stimulation *in comparison with* the results of other treatments. One could compare the effects of right hemispheric stimulation (RHS) with the results produced, for example, by bilateral hemispheric stimulation (BHS) and remedial teaching (RMT). Another point of interest would be the *surplus value* of the RHS, BHS, and RMT treatments over and above no stimulation (NS) at all. In order to make a comparison possible, the L-dyslexics can be distributed across four groups which receive the RHS, BHS, RMT, and NS treatments, respectively. Afterward one can ascertain which group turns out to be the best and also whether the best treatment is significantly better than the other treatments. In order to reach reliable conclusions concerning the effect of a treatment, still other controls are essential. It would be appropriate, for example, to utilize several therapists, each conducting a part of the RHS, BHS, and RMT treatments (obviously, no therapist is involved in the "NS treatment").

It is not possible here to mention all of the often subtle control measures that exist. The sole intent of this chapter is to give the reader some insight into the conditions that must be met in order to make a sufficiently reliable statement concerning the effects of a therapy. When conditions such as these are not met, the conclusions drawn cannot be taken seriously.

5.2. Preliminary Study

In the previous chapters, we attempted to lend credibility to the idea that the initial and advanced learning-to-read processes rest predominantly on right and left hemispheric activity, respectively. A child may get off to a wrong start by using left hemispheric strategies during initial reading; this will promote the development of a dyslexia of the L type. It may also happen that a child will become stranded after making a good start. In this case, predominantly right hemispheric strategies were used during reading, but later on *no switch* was made to left hemispheric strategies. Becoming stranded in this manner will induce the development of a dyslexia of the P type. As stated previously, the reading of L-dyslexics and P-dyslexics can be improved by stimulation of the right and left hemisphere, respectively. This kind of stimulation will change the activity of the stimulated hemisphere, and as a result, certain aspects of written language will improve.

In a nutshell, that is the essence of this book. Because the step from etiology (the cause of dyslexia) to therapy (treatment) is rather large, we decided to conduct a preliminary therapeutic study in order to ascertain whether it made sense to continue working within this therapeutic framework.

Ten L-dyslexics and nine P-dyslexics participated in this study; all were boys of 8 to 13 years of age. The L-dyslexics and P-dyslexics were each divided into three groups, containing three or four children per group. The experimental group (the E group) received hemisphere-specific stimulation—the L-dyslexics of the right, the P-dyslexics of the left hemisphere. The L-dyslexics as well as the P-dyslexics in the first control group (the C1 group) received remedial teaching, whereas the L-dyslexics and P-dyslexics in the second control group (the C2 group) were given no extra training. The E and C1 groups were trained during 16 sessions, with a duration of approximately 40 minutes per session, with one session per week.

During these sessions the L-dyslexics in the E group were given words flashed in the left visual field. These words (usually) had to be read aloud. The children were wearing headphones and could hear themselves read via the left ear. The reverse occurred in the case of the P-dyslexics in the E group: Words were flashed in the right visual field, and they could hear their own voice via the right ear. The children of the C1 group—both L-dyslexics and P-dyslexics—received remedial teaching as assigned by a special teacher. They were taken out of the classroom for this, like the children in the E group. This was not the case for L-dyslexics and P-dyslexics in the C2 group.

Various word and sentence reading tests were administered to all of the children before beginning and after completing the training sessions. In addition, the electric activity evoked by the words was recorded on the left and right sides of the skull (WRPs). The results of the reading tests were scored on accuracy (errors) and speed (number of words or sentences read). In total, 10 reading scores were obtained per child, before and after the training sessions. Each child could improve $(+)$, worsen $(-)$, or remain the same (0), on each score. *Exclusive* improvement meant 10 times a plus $(+)$ and not a single minus $(-)$ score. In this case, a child would receive a score of $+10$. And in the same fashion, exclusive worsening was indicated by a total score of -10.

Obviously more data could be given here with regard to the design and execution of this small-scale experiment. A detailed account is to be found, however, in the original publication concerning this study (Bakker, Moerland, and Goekoop-Hoefkens, 1981). Moreover, the method of hemisphere-specific stimulation (E group) does not really differ from that used in the follow-up investigation, as described in Chapter 7. With regard to the criteria used to select L-dyslexics and P-dyslexics, one is also referred to the above-mentioned publication.

The results of the preliminary study showed that hemisphere-specific stimulation influenced the activity of the right and left hemispheres of L-dyslexics and P-dyslexics, respectively, in the E group, in a manner that was not found in L-dyslexics and P-dyslexics of the C1 and C2 groups. The mean reading advantage of each group is presented in Figure 10. It is apparent that all of the groups improved on average, but the L-dyslexics and P-dyslexics in the E group showed the largest improvement (i.e., significantly greater improvement than the other groups). There were indications also that the hemisphere-specific changes in electrical brain activity were related to the improvements in reading ability.

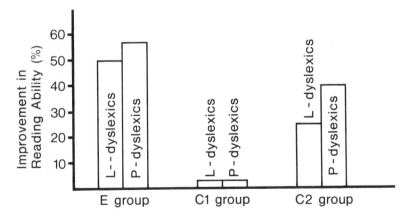

FIGURE 10. Mean percentage of improvement of reading ability in L- and P-dyslexics who received hemisphere-specific stimulation (E group) and in those who did not (C groups). (After Bakker, Moerland, & Goekoop-Hoefkens, 1981; ref. 1.)

Encouraged by these results—the fact that hemisphere-specific stimulation appeared to produce better results than other forms of treatment—we decided to continue our investigation of neuropsychological stimulation in a more extensive study.

Before embarking on a discussion of the design, execution, and results of this study, we should mention that only *significant* results will be discussed (unless stated otherwise). *Significance* is a statistical term indicating that it is highly improbable that the results obtained are due to chance.

5.3. Extensive Study

Participating in the extensive study were 35 L- and 35 P-dyslexics—55 boys and 15 girls with a mean age of 10.5 years and a mean backwardness in reading of approximately three years. The L-dyslexics made more substantive and fewer time-consuming reading errors in comparison to the P-dyslexics. On a dichotic listening test, the L-dyslexics revealed a right- and the P-dyslexics a left-ear advantage or no ear advantage. Pattern of mistakes and ear advantage were thus in accordance with the characteristics of L- and P-dyslexia as discussed earlier.

In comparison with the preliminary study, more alternative treatments were included in the extensive study. The L-dyslexics and P-dyslexics were distributed across five treatment groups: L1, L2, L3, L4, L5; and P1, P2, P3, P4, P5, respectively. L1 and P1 received hemisphere-specific stimulation, L1 of the right and P1 of the left hemisphere. This was achieved by flashing words in the left visual field of the L1 children and in the right visual field of the P1 children. The words were to be read aloud, and the vocalizations were then conducted to the left (L1) or right (P1) ear. One might have noticed that the treatment of these groups was essentially the same as that of the E group in the preliminary study.

To control for the L1 and P1 groups, L2 and P2 treatments were devised, in which words were also flashed, albeit not in the left or right, but in the central visual field. It should be recalled that in central stimulation the material is projected to both hemispheres and thus not exclusively to either the right (L1) or left hemisphere (P1). The words were flashed on a monitor and were steered by a microcomputer. To be removed from one's classroom in order to "play" with this equipment for an hour is obviously interesting and possibly also motivating. It could be that the L1 and P1 children would improve in their reading for this reason alone, and not particularly as a result of the stimulation of the right (L1) or left hemisphere (P1). Thus the L2 and P2 treatments were devised in order to show that any possible improvement in reading ability was in fact related to stimulation of the right (L1) or left (P1) hemisphere, and not to "playing" with the computer or nonspecific stimulation as such.

In the L3 and P3 groups, hemisphere-alluding stimulation of the right and left hemispheres, respectively, was employed. The children in the L3 group were given texts to read from ordinary books—ordinary except for the fact that these texts were printed in several lettertypes, all mixed up and thus perceptually complex in character. Earlier, we reasoned that perceptual complexity would activate the right hemisphere. The P3 children received the same texts, but this time everything that might increase its perceptual complexity was omitted; text was printed in a simple, very common typeface, and no colors or illustrations were included. In addition, some of the words in the text could be determined only by means of rhyming to preceding words or on the basis of text comprehension. Rhyming calls for the analysis of speech sounds and therefore makes an appeal to the left hemisphere.

L4 and P4, which were the controls for L3 and P3, respectively, received a *mixture* of the L3 and P3 treatments. Thus, L4, as well as P4, children were given texts that were sometimes perceptually laden and sometimes were not; sometimes the child had to search for (rhyme) words and sometimes did not. With respect to content, L4 and P4 were given the same texts as L3 and P3.

All of the treatments are discussed extensively in Bakker and Vinke (1985); Chapters 7 and 9 provide a more detailed description of the L1, P1, L3, and P3 treatments, including the fixation procedures used in the case of L1 and P1. On reading Chapters 7 and 9, one will learn that, for the sake of variety the L3 and P3 children performed a number of extra tasks which met the need, in these groups, of alluding to the right and left hemispheres, respectively.

L5 and P5 can be considered as "controls for the controls." The children in these groups did not receive any treatment and remained in their classrooms, whereas all of the other children were taken out of their classrooms for the treatment sessions.

The various treatments are represented schematically in Figure 11. All children (except for those in L5 and P5) were given 22 treatment sessions, each of approximately 45 minutes in duration, one session per week. Reading and spelling tests (single-word reading; sentence reading; writing to dictation) were administered before the treatments began and after their conclusion. In addition, the electric activity evoked by words (WRPs) was recorded on left and right sides of the skull.

With regard to the electrophysiological results (WRPs), we merely remark that stimulation of the right hemisphere in the L1 children and of the left hemisphere in P1 children produced effects that were not present among their immediate control groups L2 and L5, and P2 and P5, respectively. On the basis of these results and those of the preliminary studies, we can conclude that hemisphere-specific stimulation does indeed influence the activity of the stimulated hemisphere.

After the treatments, the *reading efficiency,* computed on the basis of the errors made as a percentage of the total number of words read, of the L1 children proved to have increased in comparison to the control groups (Figure 12). The same was true, although to a lesser degree, for the L3 group. The P1 group demonstrated no trace of improvement in reading efficiency, in striking contrast to the P3 and P4 groups (see Figure 12). P4 was a control group, and the improvement in reading advantage is therefore not easily accounted for. Possibly the fact that P4 received a mixture of the P3 and L3 treatments is responsible; perhaps the P3 portion of the P4 treatment brought about the increase in reading advantage.

Figure 13 shows that for the L-dyslexics, the only treatment that produced striking improvement in the dictation results was right hemisphere stimulation (L1).

From these and other results (see Bakker and Vinke, 1985), it appears that L-dyslexics who receive stimulation of the right hemisphere show particular improvement in accuracy of reading and spelling. In the case of L-dyslexics, this stimulation appears to result in a slower and more accurate style of reading and spelling.

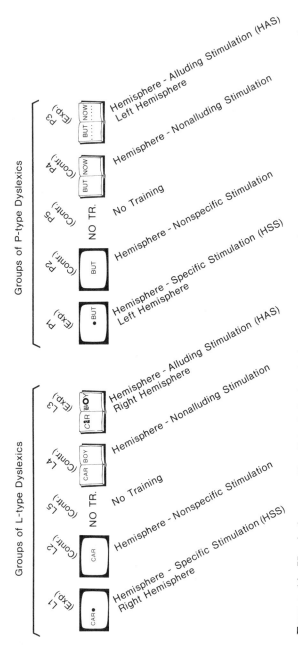

FIGURE 11. Hemisphere-specific (L1, P1), hemisphere-alluding (L3, P3), and control (L2, L4, L5, P2, P4, P5) treatments. (From Bakker & Vinke, 1985; ref. 2.)

38

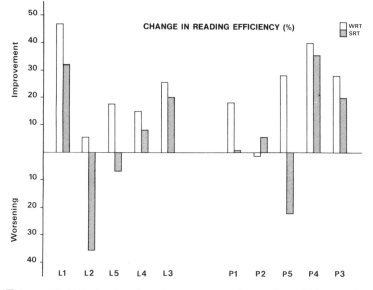

FIGURE 12. Effects of various treatments on the reading efficiency of L- and P-dyslexics. WRT, word reading test; SRT, sentence reading test. (After Bakker & Vinke, 1985; ref. 2.)

As in the preliminary investigations, electrophysiological (WRP) changes in the hemisphere were found to be related to improvements in reading ability.

It should be clear that the results of both studies indicate many similarities and few differences. With regard to reading ability, left hemispheric stimulation in P-dyslexics was effective in our preliminary study (E group) but not in our extensive study (P1). Hemisphere-alluding stimulation did prove, at least in certain respects, to be effective in P-dyslexics participating in the extensive study.

In summary, the conclusion seems justified that for L-dyslexics, right hemispheric stimulation, more than alternative treatments, is effective in ameliorating certain aspects of reading and spelling ability. It seems too early to draw reliable conclusions concerning neuropsychological treatments in P-dyslexics; we will have to wait for replication of findings.

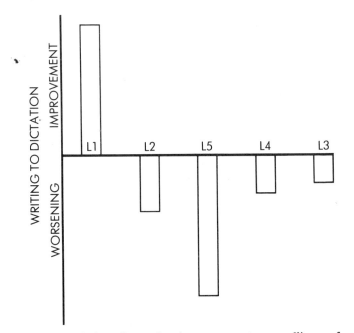

FIGURE 13. Relative effects of various treatments on spelling performance (writing to dictation) of L-dyslexics. (After Bakker & Vinke, 1985; ref. 2.)

5.4. Contributive Studies

The research to be discussed in this section does not carry much weight in and of itself, but can supplement findings that have emerged thus far concerning neuropsychological stimulation. The research referred to here has not yet been published but has been summarized in the form of reports. The significance accorded to this research is restricted by the relative inequality and small scope of the participating groups, the less than optimal control measures employed, and the limited possibilities for statistical analysis. These limitations which might apply more to one study than to another, were often inevitable on account of organizational and material constraints.

Ter Voort (1983) used hemisphere-specific stimulation in the case of three dyslexic girls of the L type. Thea, Pam, and Patty, 12, 10, and 10 years of age, respectively, received stimulation of the right hemisphere during two training periods (T1 and T2), in a manner that for all practical purposes was equivalent to the treatment received by the L1 children in the extensive study (see Sec. 5.3). Thus, words were flashed in the left visual field, and the articulations produced by the reading of these words were directed to the left ear. During the T1 and T2 periods, eight treatments of 45 minutes each were given. There were two treatment sessions per week; thus the training was more intensive than that used in the investigation discussed earlier. Preceding the T1 period—that is, during the baseline (B) period—several reading tests were administered quite a few times. This was also the case during T1 and T2, after each of the treatments. Between T1 and T2, a withdrawal (W) period was introduced, during which time no treatments were given but reading was tested (a number of times). In summary, treatments were given during the T1 and T2 periods, and reading was tested during B, T1, W, and T2, in that order.

Characteristic of this type of research is that one can examine, for each child, how the reading results obtained during the treatments relate to those of the preceding periods. The intention is, obviously, to ascertain whether the treatments have been effective.

Ter Voort speaks positively of her results:

> Evaluation of the obtained results demonstrates the import of right-hemisphere training in reading-disabled children of the L type. The girls make fewer reading errors after each training. . . . The error pattern that characterizes the L type changes in the direction of the error pattern that is characteristic of the P type—a sign that the reading-disabled child is paying more attention to the perceptual aspects of the text. At the same time, this can be seen as an indication that the subdivision in substantive and time-consuming errors is of experimental relevance. (Ter Voort, 1983, p. 66, transl.)

To illustrate these findings, Thea's results are presented in Figure 14. Notice that the number of substantive errors decreased considerably during T1, as compared to B, and increased again somewhat during W (no treatment). The second series of eight treatments (T2), once more, effectuated a decrease in the number of substantive errors. It is interesting to note that the number of

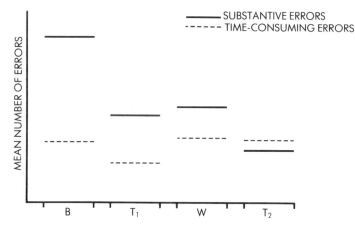

FIGURE 14. Change in the mean number of substantive and time-consuming errors made by Thea. (After Ter Voort, 1983; ref. 15.)

time-consuming errors increased across the periods and exceeded the number of substantive errors during the T2 period, As Ter Voort has suggested, the error pattern displayed by this L-dyslexic moved in the direction of the error pattern of a P-dyslexic, owing to stimulation of the right hemisphere.

The effects produced in Pam were very similar to those seen in Thea. Patty, in contrast, reacted less favorably to treatment.

A study performed by Notermans and Van de Rijdt (1984) is of interest for several reasons: first, L-dyslexics with *persistent reading problems* were treated; for these dyslexics, special educational training and/or programs that had been undertaken in the past proved to have minimal effect. Second, the efficacy of right hemisphere stimulation via the *left visual field* was compared with stimulation of that hemisphere via the *left hand*. Finally, this study is of interest because these investigators sought to determine whether stimulation of the right hemisphere affects the pattern of *eye movements* (see Chap. 2, Sec. 2.1) in the dyslexic reader. We shall comment on each of these aspects separately.

1. L-Dyslexics with persistent reading problems participated in the study. Evidently, one can assume that these children had received various treatments in the past, with no improvement. There

is a shortcoming in the research design used by Notermans and Van de Rijdt—the absence of a control group that received an alternative form of treatment or no treatment at all. Strictly speaking, one cannot ascertain, on the basis of this experiment, whether right hemispheric stimulation was successful or not. However, there is an extenuating circumstance, which is that one can assume that control treatments had already taken place in the past and that they had failed to produce a reading advantage. When viewed from this perspective, the improvement in reading after right hemispheric stimulation can be ascribed to that stimulation.

2. Up to this point in our discussion, we have not dealt with research in which the right hemisphere was stimulated by presentation of the reading material to the left hand. Chapter 8 describes the procedure that should be followed when using this method of stimulation. In this section, it is sufficient to say that in tactile or *haptic* (i.e., by touch) stimulation of the (left) hand, a "tactile training box" is used, which is constructed in such a way that the person seated behind the box can put his or her arm through the opening in the box and feel, but not see, the plastic letters lying beyond the opening. These letters can, of course, be made of materials other than plastic. The letters are fastened to a board, and when a number of such letters are used, one can construct words and sentences. The child is usually instructed to explore the letters or words by feeling their contours with one or more fingers of the hand. After the child recognizes the letters or words, he or she is asked to articulate them. A number of variations are obviously possible within this task.

3. In Chapter 2, Section 2.1, we mentioned that during reading, the eyes move from one fixation point to the next. Reading takes place during these fixations and *not* during the eye movements. The fixations and eye movements last only for a fraction of a second. Donders and Van der Vlugt (1984) have shown convincingly that P-dyslexics fixate for a relatively long period of time and produce relatively short eye movements. This is logical since P-dyslexics are particularly geared toward the shapes (perceptual characteristics) of the letters, and visual scanning of these shapes requires extra time. Notermans and Van de Rijdt (1984) utilized this concept to argue that L-dyslexics receiving right hemispheric stimulation approach the P style of reading to a certain extent, and

therefore display longer fixation times and shorter (in terms of distance and time) eye movements.

In Notermans and Van de Rijdt's experiment, the patterns of eye movements were registered with special equipment during reading, before and after the treatments (see also Spaninks & Van der Vlugt, 1981; Donders & Van der Vlugt, 1984). In addition, several reading and spelling tests were administered. A total of 16 treatments were given, two sessions per week. Stimulation of the right hemisphere was done via the left visual field (in approximately the same manner as employed in the case of the L1 group in the extensive study, discussed in Sec. 5.3) or via the left hand with the aid of the tactile training box.

On the basis of their results, the investigators concluded that

> the percentage of words read correctly has improved and the reading tempo has slowed down. It is also apparent that this training effect is maintained after the period in which no hemisphere-specific training took place. . . . The results show that the haptic training has brought about a large improvement in reading strategy and that the effect of the training is retained over a longer period of time. . . . It is apparent that the eye movements of the children of the L type have changed in the predicted direction: The mean duration of fixation has increased. . . . The effect [alterations in the pattern of eye movements] does not appear to be a lasting one because the average duration of fixation once again decreased after the period in which no hemisphere-specific training took place. . . . This training appears to be a meaningful supplement and applicable in those situations where other special educational training and/or programs have had little success. (Notermans and Van de Rijdt, 1984, p. 30, transl.)

In discussing their results, the authors mentioned a period in which no hemisphere-specific training took place. A number of months after the final treatment, the children who participated in this study were tested once again, with respect to patterns of eye movements and reading/spelling ability. This was done in order to ascertain whether the effects of treatment persisted over the interval. Results showed that the effects of treatment persisted for reading ability, but not for eye movements.

Although the conclusions of Notermans and Van de Rijdt are

encouraging, the limitations inherent in their study design must be kept in mind.

Buyle and Van Dycke (1982), as well as De Kruyk (1984), also stimulated the right hemisphere of L-type dyslexics by presenting all of the reading material to the left hands of these children. In studies by Caris and Van den Bossche (1983) and Damen (1983), P-dyslexics participated. By presenting all of the reading material to the right hand, these researchers attempted to stimulate the left hemisphere.

As all of these investigators have themselves remarked, the design of their studies is very limited or flawed. In some instances, the dyslexia subtypes were determined on the basis of varying criteria; moreover, in others, the groups used were very small, sometimes with and sometimes without control groups; in a few studies, the entire treatment involved only a limited number of sessions. Nevertheless, these studies are of value in that some of them provide considerable detail on how the haptic treatment was carried out and how the children reacted to it. The treatment of two children, an L-dyslexic and a P-dyslexic, carried out by Damen, is illustrative in this respect. However tentative their conclusions, these researchers are moderately or even considerably optimistic regarding the value of hemisphere-specific stimulation via the hands. This type of stimulation was found to be more effective for L-dyslexics than for P-dyslexics, although some success was demonstrated even in the latter group.

5.5. Recent Studies

After the original publication of this text in Dutch, other investigations into the effects of hemisphere-specific stimulation were initiated. As a first step in replicating our findings, Grace (1987), at the University of Victoria in Canada, used hemisphere-specific stimulation in three dyslexic children—one L type and two P types. Three other children, two L-dyslexics and one P-dyslexic, served as controls. All of the children attended a summer school program. The children who received hemisphere-specific stimulation were treated for 12 sessions, three sessions per week. Letters and words were flashed in the left visual field of the L-dyslexic in order to stimulate the right hemisphere, and in the right visual field of the P-dyslexics in order to stimulate the left hemisphere. Reading, spelling, and arithmetic, among other skills, were pre- and post-tested in all subjects. Before and after the treatments, WRPs to centrally flashed words were recorded at right and left temporal and parietal locations. Thus, the design of Grace's pilot investigation and that of our preliminary and extensive studies were quite similar. Furthermore, Grace reported that the results of her study paralleled those of our investigations. As compared to controls, her L-dyslexic made fewer substantive errors during reading, whereas her P-dyslexics made fewer time-consuming errors. Moreover, the children who received treatment, as compared to the untreated ones, demonstrated the predicted changes in hemispheric activity (parietal P320 amplitudes). Grace's findings, while encouraging, are only preliminary, and the results of a more extensive and sophisticated study are pending.

Not very long ago, another study was conducted because about 60 remedial teachers from all parts of the Netherlands expressed an interest in treating their dyslexic pupils with hemisphere-specific stimulation, using the tactile training box. After a reading test was administered to all of these children, the number of substantive and time-consuming errors was registered. Children who made more than the average number of substantive errors and an average, or less than average, number of time-consuming errors were considered to be L-dyslexics, whereas children who made more than an average number of time-consuming errors and an average, or less than average, number of substantive errors were considered to be P-dyslexics. All together, 98 children could be classified into L and P types. The L-dyslexics were divided into experimental and control groups, as were the P-dyslexics. The experimental and control children did not differ with regard to mean age, mean reading age, sex, and hand preference. The experimental L- and P-type dyslexics received hemisphere-specific stimulation with all of the reading material, out of sight, being presented to the fingers of the left hand in L types and to the fingers of the right hand in P types (plastic letters were used, which were fastened to a board). There were 20 sessions of approximately 45 minutes each, two sessions per week. The letters, words, and sentences that were used had to be adapted to the individual child's reading level. The control children were treated according to the discretion of the remedial teachers. All children were pre- and posttested with, for example, a word-reading and a sentence-reading test. These tests were administered also after half of the treatments had been given—that is, after 10 treatment sessions. This study may be viewed as a *field experiment*—that is, an investigation that lacks many of the strict methodological controls that characterize a *laboratory experiment*. For instance, the control treatments devised by the remedial teachers probably varied from one remedial teacher to the other, as did the operationalizations of our request to stimulate the experimental subjects with reading material at a level adequate for each child. Factors such as this may have introduced random variations within the treatment groups. It is very encouraging, therefore, that after treatment (1) the L-dyslexics showed more improvement with respect to accuracy of sentence reading (i.e., fewer substantive errors) than did the control L-dyslexics, and (2) the experimental P-dyslexics, as compared to their controls, showed more improvement with respect to fluency of word reading (fewer time-consuming errors). That the greatest improvements were achieved midway through the treatment program (10th session), with a leveling off thereafter, is a finding that merits further reflection.

A third, recently completed investigation consists of two single-case studies (Bakker, Van Leeuwen, and Spyer, 1987). One L- and one P-type dyslexic boy completed five experimental phases: (1) baseline, (2) placebo, and (3) piracetam (see below), followed by (4) piracetam + hemisphere-specific stimulation, and, once again, (5) piracetam. Reading performance was tested several times during each of these periods. A total of twelve 30-minute sessions of hemisphere-specific stimulation were given via the fingers of the left and right hand in the L- and the P-dyslexic, respectively. Piracetam* is a nootropic drug which has been reported to facilitate reading, especially speed of reading, and to affect word-related brain potentials (WRPs), predominantly in the left hemisphere (Bakker, Wilsher, Debruyne, and Bertin, 1987). In view of these effects on the speed of reading and activity of the left hemisphere, it was predicted that piracetam would have a positive

---

* 2-Oxo-1-pyrrolidineacetamide; tradenames: Euvifor, Gabacet, Genogris, Nootron, Nootropyl, Normabrain, Pirroxil.

effect on the reading of the P-type, rather than the L-type dyslexic boy. It was also predicted that hemisphere-specific stimulation would add significantly to the impact of piracetam in the P-dyslexic. In support of these hypotheses, piracetam was demonstrated to improve the reading performance of the P-dyslexic, but not that of the L-dyslexic. It was also found that hemisphere-specific stimulation significantly enhanced the piracetam effect in the P-dyslexic. That the same treatment brought about a differential effect in L- and P-type dyslexics supports the validity of the L/P classification (see also Chap. 3, Sec. 3.3).

5.6. Concluding Remarks

When we examine the results of all of the studies discussed thus far, it is quite apparent that the most striking result is the beneficial effect of right hemisphere stimulation in L-dyslexics. Not a single investigation has yielded results contradicting this conclusion. Positive results were achieved predominantly in L-dyslexics who received visual stimulation of the right hemisphere via the left visual field. Similar results were obtained with haptic stimulation via the left hand. The current state of our knowledge does not permit us to say, with certainty, which hemisphere-specific treatment, visual or haptic, is preferable.

The concordant results obtained with specific stimulation of the right hemisphere can be viewed even more optimistically when one considers that the effects of this treatment were compared with the results of alternative treatments. Thus we examined the merits of hemisphere-specific stimulation not only as compared to *no* treatment, but also as compared to other kinds of therapies. Of course, one should keep in mind that hemisphere-specific stimulation in L-dyslexics has not been compared to *all* existing alternative treatments. It is, in principle, possible that certain therapies could have a demonstrable effect in L-dyslexics that would be superior to that of specific stimulation of the right hemisphere.

Additional conclusions can also be drawn. For example, in those studies in which girls participated, there were no sex differences in the results obtained with hemisphere-specific stimulation. Furthermore, of particular interest was the finding that this treatment appeared to be beneficial for those L-dyslexics who had responded poorly, if at all, to other treatments.

One may thus conclude that right-hemisphere stimulation benefits L-dyslexics. However, its efficacy is not maximal, and it fails to ameliorate *all* aspects of written language ability. That the efficacy of the treatment is not maximal means that the treatment will not transform a dyslexic reader into a normal reader. However, probably no one really expected such an ideal result. That the treatment does not affect all aspects of written language is exemplified by the fact that stimulation of the right hemisphere in L-dyslexics does not necessarily improve their speed of reading; in other words, they are not necessarily capable of reading more words. In fact, the opposite appears to be true: L-dyslexics read more slowly on account of the treatment, possibly owing to an increase in the amount of attention given to the perceptual characteristics of the text. As a result, probably fewer errors are made, with the net outcome being an improvement in reading efficiency. These same factors probably are responsible for the increase in accuracy during writing to dictation. Some caution is needed, however, when one is attempting to draw conclusions with regard to spelling (writing to dictation.) Only one study demonstrated that right hemispheric stimulation improves spelling ability in L-dyslexics (see Sec. 5.3), but in this study the result was clear and irrefutable.

Is a dyslexic of the P type helped by receiving hemisphere-specific stimulation of the left hemisphere? Such stimulation did help in the initial, preliminary study (Sec. 5.2): P-dyslexics who received left hemispheric stimulation via the right visual field made improvements in reading ability.

The effects of haptic stimulation of the left hemisphere via the right hand have not been investigated extensively. Caris and Van den Bossche (1983) reported a trend toward increased reading speed, accompanied by an increase in the number of words correctly read, in three P-dyslexics who received haptic treatment. The latter result was also obtained by Damen (1983), in a P-type boy whom she had treated. Interestingly enough, Damen, as well as Caris and Van den Bossche, reported a decrease in the number of time-consuming errors, whereas the field experiment with the remedial teachers revealed a similar effect in P-dyslexic children.

A decrease in the number of time-consuming errors would indeed be expected when the left hemisphere of P-dyslexics is stimulated.

We should again allude to the results, discussed in Section 5.3, of our extensive study: Specific stimulation of the left hemisphere in P-dyslexics was of no avail. Therefore, one must conclude that overall, left hemispheric stimulation via the right visual field has, thus far, yielded some but not uniformly positive results. Left hemispheric stimulation via the right hand, rather than via the right visual field, seems most beneficial in P-type dyslexia.

Hemisphere-alluding stimulation in L- and P-type dyslexia has proved to be beneficial in the cases investigated (see Sec. 5.3). Especially in P-dyslexia, it appears that reading efficiency improved after *alluding stimulation* of the left hemisphere (see below). Thus, dyslexics of this type *appear* to profit from rhyming and other exercises that allude to the left hemisphere. The use of the word "appears" is deliberate since a more final evaluation will be possible only when the results of replication studies are known.

Alluding stimulation of the right hemisphere—that is, stimulation by means of perceptually laden script—appears to have a positive effect on the reading efficiency of L-type dyslexics (see Sec. 5.3). There is, however, no indication that spelling ability improves as a result of this treatment. One will recall that it did improve in the case of hemisphere-specific stimulation of the right hemisphere—a treatment that proved to yield the largest improvement in L-dyslexics with regard to reading.

Given the present state of these investigations, we recommend the following:

1. Treat dyslexics of the L type with hemisphere-specific stimulation of the right hemisphere, either via the left visual field (preferably) or via the left hand.
2. As an alternative, treat dyslexics of the L type with hemisphere-alluding stimulation of the right hemisphere.
3. Treat dyslexics of the P type with hemisphere-specific stimulation of the left hemisphere, preferably via the right hand.
4. As a possible alternative, treat dyslexics of the P type with hemisphere-alluding stimulation of the left hemisphere.

One could also investigate whether it is beneficial to alternate treatments 1 and 2 in L-dyslexics and treatments 3 and 4 in P-dyslexics.

6

Important Questions

6.1. Questions of Theoretical Import

Research yields not only answers but also questions, not in the least in the investigator him- or herself. This chapter explores questions that have been asked or that could be asked. We should state in advance that it is not possible to answer all of these questions definitively. It is nevertheless essential to pose these questions and to attempt to find answers through research. Some of these problems are, at present, predominantly of theoretical import, but certainly today's theory can shape tomorrow's practice.

One question that has been posed addresses what happens in the brain when hemisphere-specific and -alluding stimulation are applied. It is now evident that the pattern of electric activity changes and that this change is related to improvements in reading and spelling ability. The brain functions in systems that can be conceived as complex electrical and chemical circuits, with the chains of connecting nerve cells being the "wiring." Each type of behavior has a corresponding circuit to which it relates more than to another circuit. It is possible that certain circuits that are important in reading are not readily "passable," and, as a consequence, the learning-to-read process is impeded. Perhaps the effect of stimulation is to lower those "thresholds" that are exceedingly high in these circuits so that during reading, important information can be transmitted more swiftly. The main problem is, of course, to locate these circuits.

At present, one can only speculate on the nature of these circuits. Authorities in the field have, more than once, suggested that (hemisphere-specific?) circuits regulating attentional processes (arousal) may be involved. This hypothesis is currently under investigation in our laboratory. In the event of a positive result, the attention factor could be integrated into the therapeutic regimen.

It may also be that hemisphere-specific stimulation enhances the "interhemispheric exchange" of information. An example might suffice to explain this rather complicated phrase. Imagine an L-dyslexic whose right hemisphere is being stimulated via the left visual field. The words (i.e., the information) are projected to the right hemisphere. From there, the information spreads to other parts of the brain—among others, to the left hemisphere—mainly via the corpus callosum. It has been suggested that this kind of interhemispheric exchange will lead to an improvement in reading ability. If this theory proves to be valid, methods should be designed to take advantage of this transfer of information from the one hemisphere to the other. In this case, alterations of the hemisphere-specific and -alluding treatment methods could probably be achieved in order to attain this goal.

Another question concerns why one dyslexic child develops into an L-dyslexic, and another into a P-dyslexic, and whether certain reading methods play a role in their differential development. Regretfully, at this time it is not possible to provide a satisfactory answer to these questions; however, we can say that their import lies in the fact that they stimulate reflection on the *prevention* of dyslexia. With the goal of prevention in mind, one could look for signs of a (functional) overdevelopment of one of the hemispheres during the kindergarten stage in children who are "at risk" dyslexics, and subsequently devise strategies aimed at restoring the balance in hemispheric activity. To put it another way, one could apply hemisphere-specific and/or -alluding stimulation in preschoolers who are at risk of developing dyslexia, with the intention of warding off the threat of dyslexia.

For example, some prevention-oriented research was carried out recently in England by Bradley and Bryant (1985). These investigators are of the conviction that mastery of what they call the "phonological analysis of words" is an important prerequisite for the normal development of the learning-to-read process. Phonological abilities can be trained by means of rhymes. Bradley and Bryant gave rhyme exercises to children attending kindergarten who were at risk of developing dyslexia. After moving on to elementary school, those children who had been given exercises in kindergarten were indeed shown to have better reading performance than those who had not received the exercises in kindergarten. Suppose that the trained children, who were successful in elementary school, were largely "latent" P types at the time that they were attending kindergarten. In that case, one could say that these preschoolers had been treated in the same manner and just as successfully as the "acute" P types, who received comparable rhyme exercises in the extensive study (Chap. 5, Sec. 5.3). However, it is not known whether the Bradley and Bryant at-risk preschoolers were of the latent P type. Nevertheless, irrespective of whether parallels can be drawn between the Bradley and Bryant study and our L/P research, it is important to mention this study to show that preventing dyslexia is an important and workable option.

Whereas the development of a P-type dyslexia is readily conceivable, even on the basis of intuition alone, the development of L-dyslexia is not so comprehensible. L-dyslexics are believed to make use predominantly of linguistic strategies during reading, owing to premature activation of these strategies during the learning-to-read process. One could conclude, on the basis of L-type development, that L-dyslexics are linguistically skilled. Undoubtedly, upon further reflection, one would have to reexamine this conclusion, because dyslexics who are skilled in (spoken) language are few and far between! In actuality, L-dyslexics are not necessarily skilled linguistically. Rather, they are "linguistically zealous": (Spoken) Language dominates, but domination and effectiveness are quite different properties.

At this point, it seems appropriate to point out that the L/P classification is in accord with classifications of the dyslexias proposed by other investigators. Since the early 1980s, subtyping of learning disabilities has frequently been employed, and a book has even been published which deals solely with this topic (Rourke, 1985).

6.2. Questions of Practical Import

Somewhat disconcerting is the question, posed every so often, as to whether the neuropsychological treatments that have been described are more effective than other forms of remediation. Unfortunately, this question cannot be answered because, in our study, comparisons were made with several, but not all, alternative treatment methods. For that reason, it is essential to undertake more (*controlled*) comparative research.

Do the effects of the treatments last? Although this is a very important question, it can be answered only inadequately at present because the meagre information that exists was gathered informally. Notermans and Van de Rijdt (1984), investigating whether the effect of hemisphere-specific treatment was still present after a school vacation of approximately two months, found that the effect had not disappeared. Damen (personal communication) reached a similar conclusion when she retested her two dyslexics after the summer break. The reader will recall that in the three L-dyslexic girls who were treated by Ter Voort (1983), reading ability declined somewhat, although not greatly, during the W phase, the period in which no treatment was given. These findings suggest that the effects do *last* over a period of a number of weeks. However, more research, is needed to determine whether this conclusion is correct. At present, nothing can be said with respect to the effects over the long term.

Again in regard to treatment effects, for how long and how intensively must one treat before an effect is noticeable? Does the magnitude of the effect increase linearly with the length of treatment? These are important questions which, regrettably, cannot really be addressed on the basis of the data now at hand. For purely organizational reasons, treatment, in the research carried out until now, was given once or twice a week (Grace treated her children three times a week), in sessions lasting 45 minutes at most. Never have more than 22 sessions been given. It would, in all respects, be worthwhile to investigate the relationship between *duration* and *intensity of treatment,* on the one hand, and *treatment effect,* on the other.

In regard to the relationship between treatment duration and treatment effect, one might recall that 22 treatment sessions were given in the course of our extensive study (Chap. 5, Sec. 5.3). Before, as well as after, the sessions, reading and other tests were administered. In addition, a reading test was administered once every two months during the treatment period. If one were to plot the

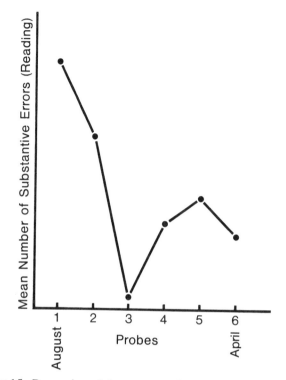

FIGURE 15. Regression of the mean number of substantive reading errors in L1-dyslexics (L1 group; see Fig. 11) over a treatment period of approximately nine months. (After Reitsma, 1985; ref. 12.)

number of errors on this reading test, for L-dyslexics who received hemisphere-specific stimulation, versus the duration of treatment, then a graph like that shown in Figure 15 would be obtained.

Statistical (trend) analysis shows that (1) the number of reading errors decreased linearly with the number of treatment sessions given, suggesting that the longer an individual is treated, the more accurate his or her reading becomes; but also that (2) after a certain number of treatments, no more improvement can be expected. To avoid any misinterpretation, it is important to emphasize that Figure 15 refers to the *hemisphere-specific* treatment of L-dyslexics (group L1; see Chap. 5, Sec. 5.3). Other (control) treatments revealed either a different course in the number of reading errors, or none at all (Reitsma, 1985). In this connection, the field experiment (see Chap. 5, Sec. 5.5) produced an interesting result: The improvement of reading accuracy in the experimental L-dyslexics was largest after 10 treatment sessions, with a leveling off thereafter. Similarly, the decrease in number of time-consuming errors in the experimental P-dyslexics was largest after 10 treatment sessions. It is tempting to speculate on the mechanism for the nonlinear trends in both the extensive study and the field experiment. One might propose that children initially are highly motivated to read because of the novelty of the computer screen or tactile training box and that this motivation levels off after a number of treatments. Motivation may initially cause reading performance to improve, whereas habituation may subsequently arrest the improvement. However, this explanation is at variance with the finding that other dyslexic children who also received computer-aided treatment (e.g., the L2, P2, and P1 treatment groups in the extensive study; see Chap. 5, Sec. 5.3), did not improve at all. An interesting suggestion was advanced by one of my students, who reminded me of evidence that the relationship between degree of arousal and mental performance is U-shaped: Moderate arousal is initially accompanied by improvement in mental performance, but excessive arousal leads to a decrease in performance. Is it possible that reading improvement is associated with a moderate, rather than an excessive, increase of hemisphere-specific arousal over the course of the treatment sessions? For a pertinent discussion of the possible association between arousal modulations and cognitive proficiency, one is referred to the study by Morris (1989). Yet another mechanism may account for the finding that reading improvement in some of our studies tended to level off after a number of treatments. Learning curves generally are asymptotic, and therefore the learning of reading by dyslexics who have received treatment may only be reflecting the norm. If this is the case, then perhaps the leveling off could be prevented by the introduction of a new treatment at some point: For example, hemisphere-alluding stimulation could follow hemisphere-specific stimulation, or vice versa. More research is needed to shed some light on these questions.

We have repeatedly mentioned the concepts of treatment, stimulation, and training. One may wonder what the dyslexic child, who is being submitted to this treatment, thinks of it. Some investigators, Damen (1983) as well as others, have noted their impressions. In general, the treatments appear to be regarded as pleasant, especially in the beginning. This is quite understandable, for, after all, the child is allowed to "play" with computers and tactile training boxes! The novelty of it does, however, wear off over the long run, and occasionally, albeit not often, the initial interest turns into boredom. There is an impression (but not more than that) that the fun lasted somewhat longer in the case of haptic stimulation by way of the tactile training box, than in the case of visual stimulation via computer and monitor, perhaps because the tasks given during haptic stimulation were quite varied. Whatever the case may be, it is an important issue that concerns the educational design of the treatments. With respect to all variation considered necessary in the therapy, the only restriction is that one must remain within the framework of hemisphere-specific or -alluding stimulation, at least if one wishes to do justice to the methods of neuropsychological treatment of dyslexia that have been presented. To master these schemata, it is essential to examine the scientific sources upon which this book is based. Experience and common sense will have to do the rest.

Hemisphere-Specific
Stimulation (HSS)
via the Visual Half-Fields

7.1. Overview

The trainee (TE) is seated, at a distance of approximately 90 cm, in front of the monitor (M), which is connected to a microcomputer; TE is looking at the space between two dots, placed one above the other, in the middle of M. TE's chair is adjustable vertically, and the two dots are located at eye level. TE is wearing headphones which are connected to a stereo tape recorder. A microphone, connected to the headphones, has been placed directly in front of TE. The index finger of TE's dominant hand is held directly above the reaction knob (RK), located on the switchboard (SB). The entire setup is illustrated in Figure 16.

If TE is a dyslexic of the L type, the following will happen: While TE is staring at the space between the dots on M, a third dot will appear in that space. As soon as TE sees this third dot, he or she will press the RK, on the SB, as quickly as possible. The pressing of RK triggers the flashing of a word (*a*) or two words (*b*) to the left of the two dots—that is, in the left visual field (LVF)—and simultaneously with this, a star (*) will (*c*) or will not (*d*) appear to the right of the two dots—that is, in the right visual field (RVF). When both *a* and *c* occur, TE is supposed to say the word aloud, and subsequently say "yes." By saying "yes," TE acknowledges the fact that a star was present. If *a* and *d* occur, TE should say the word aloud and say "no" (i.e., there was no star) afterward. When two words are presented (*b*), these

copy

rectholosy

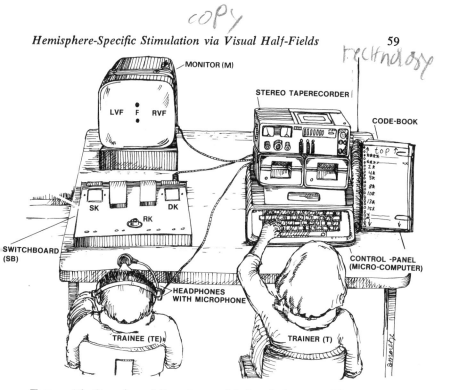

FIGURE 16. Overview of the setup used in hemisphere-specific treatment via the visual half-fields; F, place where the fixation dot will appear; LVF, left visual field; RVF, right visual field; RK, reaction knob; SK, same knob; DK, different knob. The *g, f, r, c,* and *s* keys are located on the control panel of the microcomputer (see Chap. 7, Sec. 7.4).

words are of equal length and placed one above the other. If *b* occurs, and the two words are, according to TE, the same, then TE will press the "same knob" (SK) on the SB. If TE, however, considers the words to be different, then he or she will press the "different knob" (DK) on the SB. Thus *b* always coincides with *c* or with *d.* For the combination *b–c,* TE presses SK or DK and says "yes" (there was a star). For the combination *b–d,* TE presses SK or DK and says "no" (there was no star).

When pronouncing the words (*a*) and saying "yes" or "no," TE will hear, via the microphone and headphones, his or her own

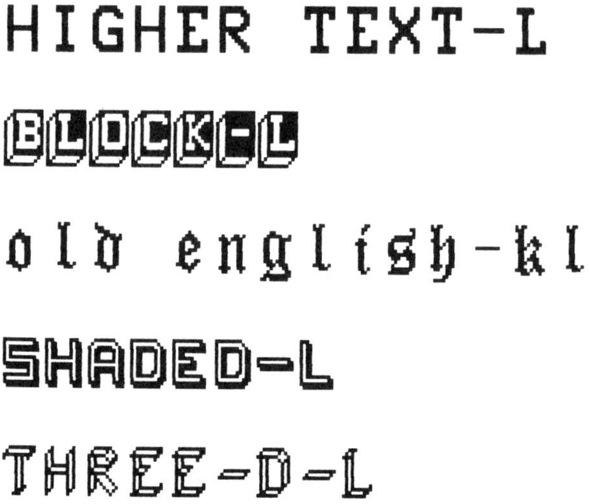

HIGHER TEXT-L

BLOCK-L

old english-kl

SHADED-L

THREE-D-L

FIGURE 17. Letter types of words flashed in the case of the L-dyslexic (synergistic software).

voice in the left ear. The voice of the trainer also will be heard by TE in the left ear, via the same route. Via the tape recorder, TE will hear light, nonvocal music in the right ear.

The words presented to TE in the LVF appear at an angle of 2.5–5.0° and refer, in terms of meaning, to a concrete object. The lettertypes are perceptually demanding (types: higher text; Old English; shaded-L; block; three-dimensional; see Figure 17).

A dyslexic of the P type will follow the same procedure as the L-type dyslexic, with these exceptions: A single word (*a;* thus never two words) is flashed (at an angle of 2.5–5.0°) to the right (RVF) of the central dots. The appearance of that word is (*c*) or is not (*d*) accompanied by the presentation of a star to the left (LVF) of the dots. TE's task is to (*a1*) say the word aloud or, (*a2*) first spell the word phonetically (foreward or backward), and then pronounce it. Both *a1* and *a2* are combined with *c* ("yes") or *d* ("no"). Afterward, the trainer may elicit the sequential position held by a letter in the word TE has just phonetically pronounced. TE will subsequently answer "first," "second," or "third," etc., and will then, once again, pronounce the word in its entirety.

The trainer may also, arbitrarily, pronounce a letter phonetically and then ask whether this letter appeared in the word. TE will answer "yes" or "no" and will, once again, pronounce the word.

During the execution of all tasks, TE hears his or her own voice, as well as that of the trainer, in the right ear, while light, nonvocal music is being heard in the left ear. The words, which are presented to TE on the monitor, have a more or less abstract meaning and the lettertypes are perceptually "neutral" (lower-case, small-roman type).

7.2. Fixation Procedure

In the preceding section, we stated that once the reaction knob (RK) is pressed, a word (or words) will appear on the left (L-dyslexics) or right (P-dyslexics) side of monitor M. It should be mentioned, however, that this occurs only if the *reaction time* (REAT) proves to be smaller than the *reference time* (REFT). REFT is determined *before the actual treatment is begun.* To determine REFT, TE is seated in front of the monitor, in exactly the same manner as in the actual treatment later on. In the middle of M, two dots are present, and the trainer informs TE that very soon a third dot (fixation dot) will appear between the two dots already present. TE is requested to react as quickly as possible to the emergence of the third dot by pressing RK with the index finger of the dominant hand. Subsequently, the third (fixation) dot will reappear again and again (for a total of 10 times), with arbitrary intervals ranging from 100 to 1000 ms; TE will react to all of these by pressing RK as quickly as possible. TE's mean reaction time, called REFT, is then rounded off to one of the following values: 300, 350, 400, 450, 500, 550, 600, 700, 800, or 900 ms. During the treatment, a word (or words) is flashed, left or right on M, only if TE's reaction to the fixation dot is faster than (or equal to) TE's previously determined REFT. If TE's reaction is slower, then instead of a word (or words) being flashed, a tone is heard. TE is subsequently told that he or she can react more quickly by looking carefully at the space between the dots on the middle of M. If, during the treatment, TE fails more than nine times per set of 20 word presentations, then the REFT is raised (from 350 to 400 ms, for example). If TE fails only once or not at all during a set, then the REFT is lowered (from 350 to 300 ms, for example). At the start of a treatment session, the REFT is adjusted to that with which TE ended the previous session. The aim of the REFT procedure is to effectuate fixation of the central dot. When the reaction to the fixation dot lasts longer than REFT, then TE was possibly not looking carefully at the middle of M, that is, not fixating. Not fixating should be avoided.

The star (*) which, during the treatment, may appear in the RVF (in the case of L-dyslexics) or in the LVF (in the case of P-dyslexics), simultaneously with the flashing of a word (words) in the other visual field, serves as yet another control on fixation. The star will appear 10 times per set of 20 word presentations. Which word presentation is to be accompanied by a star is determined arbitrarily so that TE is uncertain whether it will be present or absent during every word flash. The star is, however, never present or absent more than three times in succession. The chances of giving a *correct answer*—that is, the correct perception of the word (words) in the one field and of the presence/absence of a star in the other—are the greatest when TE looks at the fixation dot during the presentation.

That the fixation procedure is rather laborious, and its programing quite time-consuming is obvious. For this reason, more simple but equally reliable procedures have been sought. Dr. Robin Morris (personal communication) of Atlanta has devised the following alternative: A dot is permanently present in the middle of M, and there is also a movable dot somewhere else on M. By means of a "joystick," TE will transport the movable dot to the middle of M. As soon as the two dots merge, a word (words) will be flashed to the left (in the case of L-dyslexics) or to the right (in the case of P-dyslexics) of the dot. In this manner, TE has practically no other choice but to focus on the dot in the middle of M. We say "practically" no other choice because theoretically TE could look to the left or the right and try to merge the two dots by chance. A "hit-or-miss" approach such as this will require a lot of time, however, so that the trainer will immediately be able to correct TE's method. Some experience has already been acquired with the joystick and we found that children enjoy this method.

7.3. Choice of Words and Duration of Presentation

For the treatment of L-type dyslexia, words are flashed in the LVF, whereas in P-type dyslexia the presentation of words takes place in the RVF. A word (pair) is never presented for longer than 300 ms. If the duration of presentation were longer, TE would still have the opportunity to move his or her eyes away from the middle to the left or to the right. At the onset of a treatment, a word (pair) is shown for 300 ms. The presentation duration is lowered once TE makes no more than two errors per set of 20 word presentations and raised if more than 10 errors are made. Possible presentation times are 20, 30, 40, 50, 70, 100, 150, 200, 250, and 300 ms. At the start of a session, the presentation time is adjusted to that with which TE ended the previous session. If it appears that TE has to get acclimated once again, then the next highest value of presentation time is instituted.

Word (pairs) are presented in sets of 20. The length of the words varies from one to four letters, and the degree of difficulty has three levels. Examples of words that were used in the treatment of L- and P-dyslexics are shown in Figure 18. Figure 19 presents a complete set of words to be used for P-dyslexics, as well as a set of word pairs to be used for L-dyslexics. Several sets are available for each word length or level of difficulty. Usually several sets of equal word length and level of difficulty are used during one treatment session.

7.4. Treatment Procedure

The trainer inputs TE's profile (name, type, grade, etc.) into the computer and retrieves the suitable program from the computer's memory. The trainer sits beside TE and has the keyboard of the computer as well as a list of words (codebook) in front of him- or herself. The list consists of the words (word pairs) that TE will be seeing on the screen. The list is comprised of 20 words or word pairs. Next to each word/word pair on the list, a star is either present or absent so that the trainer can easily see what TE is

Example of concrete words used (L-dyslexics):

Degree of difficulty 1: 1 letter*: i,h,d,l,z,e,c,w,j,k,e,f
                        2 letters: po,wy,pa,ar,ui,me,ei,ze,jy,el,eg,la
                        3 letters: dop,bel,bal,pit,tor,zon,mat,hok,vat,lip,roe
                        4 letters: haan,soep,kool,nier,tuin,room,meer,kuit,veer

Degree of difficulty 2: 3 letters: pyl,mok,kap,zak,kip,vis,wol,eik,dyk,zag,pek
                        4 letters: neus,zool,zaag,teil,huid,kuif,gier,haas,mama

Degree of difficulty 3: 3 letters: jam,wak,lyn,rad,oma,map,pon,wyf,juk,aar,ven
                        4 letters: blad,fles,balk,park,ster,lamp,tree,klok,snor

---

* Single letters were used for those children who were incapable of reading 2-
or 3-letter words.

Example of abstract words used (P-dyslexics):

Degree of difficulty 1: 1 letter*: y,o,u,r,s,p,h,i,j,g,l,k
                        2 letters: by,ha,pi,ho,om,of,do,mi,uk,is,yl,ga
                        3 letters: uur,nul,net,pas,bar,min,tel,nog,met,mee,rap
                        4 letters: deel,vier,week,maar,poos,zaal,reis,voor,tien

Degree of difficulty 2: 3 letters: gul,fyn,zin,aai,ons,oer,bof,wit,pyn,rui,tof
                        4 letters: zaak,toon,lied,goor,taak,raar,neen,boel,rein

Degree of difficulty 3: 3 letters: muf,lui,hof,fut,ruw,wie,nop,erf,ene,alt,ryp
                        4 letters: land,gaaf,klap,kans,druk,stop,rand,zoet,slim

FIGURE 18. Examples of Dutch words used for L- and P-dyslexics.

supposed to say or do after each presentation. After the treatment procedure is operational, TE will give either a vocal response (naming) or a manual response (pressing SK or DK when two words are presented). Manual responses are automatically recorded by the computer as correct or incorrect. In the case of a correct vocal response, the trainer presses the *g* (GOOD) key on the keyboard, after which the next word will appear. The *f* (FAILURE) key is pressed when a vocal answer is incorrect. By subsequently pressing the *r* (REPEAT) key, the word in question will reappear with a presentation time of 300 ms. If the answer given

Set C-3-2-20-2*	Set A-4-1-20-2**
zee-hak	keer
vla-mok	leen
das-byl	neer
hak-hak	niet
sla-rok	maat
wol-wol	vaak
wei-wei	beet
arm-arm	goed
bok-dak	beet
zee-zee	geel
vos-vel	toen
bed-lym	goed
rol-rol	tien
rug-rug	hoek
vel-vel	poos
alp-lap	leeg
dak-dak	beet
pek-lap	boos
kap-kap	naar
aas-kei	gaan

*C =	concrete	**A =	abstract
3 =	three letters	4 =	four letters
2 =	degree of difficulty	1 =	degree of difficulty
20 =	20 word pairs	20 =	20 words
2 =	set no. 2	2 =	set no. 2

FIGURE 19. Example of a complete set of (the original Dutch) word pairs used for L-dyslexics (C-3-2-20-2) and a complete set of words for P-dyslexics (A-4-1-20-2).

this time is correct, then the trainer will press the *c* (CONTINUE) key. If the answer is, once again, incorrect, then the *s* (SHOW) key is pressed; the word in question will then reappear and stay on the screen. In this case the trainer will say, "That was not correct; we will look and see what it really says." The reading is helped along, if necessary. Afterward, the procedure is continued by pressing the *c* key. The *s* key is not used more than five times during a set of 20 words (pointing out errors more often than this might discourage TE).

A session lasts for 30–45 min, and generally no more than five word sets will be utilized during this time. If a child is quick (few fixation errors; few errors during word reading), one can, if necessary or desired, continue with the first set of that session, after the presentation of five sets. Before the treatment takes place, the trainer must be very familiar with the microcomputer program and the word lists that TE will be given. On these lists (sets), the words accompanied by a star have been marked; the trainer asks TE to give the sequential position (first, second, third, or fourth) of the underlined letters. Figure 20 provides an overview of treatment across 20 sessions.

In summary, the following occurs during the course of a treatment:

1. TE is seated in front of M and is given headphones to wear which are connected to a tape recorder.
2. The tape recorder is switched on.
3. TE is given instructions on the task and is requested to look closely at the center of M.
4. The trainer presses the key that activates the program.
5. If TE presses the knob on time, the first word will appear. If the child is late, he or she will hear a beep and will have to fixate once again.
6. TE responds (either vocally or manually).
7. If the answer is correct, the trainer will press the key for the next word. If the answer is incorrect, the trainer will press the key for repetition of the word. If the answer given now is correct, then the trainer will press the key for the next word. If the answer is once again incorrect, then he or she will press the key that keeps the word on the screen. TE will now give the answer, if necessary with the aid of the trainer (a correction is given a maximum of five times during one set). The trainer will now press the key for the following word.
8. After a set of words has been completed, the trainer will, depending on TE's performance, look at the results together with TE and, if necessary, adjust the fixation time and/or presentation time.

	L-type				P-type			
Session	Letter type	Word type	Task	No.of words	Letter type	Word type	Task	No.of words
1	HT	C2-1	M	2	RK	A2-1	N	1
2	HT	C2-1	M	2	RK	A2-1	N	1
3	HT	C3-1	N	1	RK	A3-1	N	1
4	HT	C3-1	N	1	RK	A3-1	N	1
5	TD	C4-1	N	1	RK	A4-1	N	1
6	TD	C4-1	N	1	RK	A4-1	N	1
7	TD	C3-2	M	2	RK	A3-2	Sf	1
8	TD	C3-2	M	2	RK	A3-2	Sf	1
9	BL	C4-2	N	1	RK	A4-2	Ra	1
10	BL	C4-2	N	1	RK	A4-2	Ra	1
11	BL	C3-3	N	1	RK	A3-3	Rb	1
12	BL	C3-3	N	1	RK	A3-3	Rb	1
13	SH	C4-3	M	2	RK	A4-3	N	1
14	SH	C4-3	M	2	RK	A4-3	N	1
15	SH	C2-1	N	1	RK	A2-1	Sb	1
16	SH	C2-1	N	1	RK	A2-1	Sb	1
17	OE	C3-1	N	1	RK	A3-1	Ra	1
18	OE	C4-1	N	1	RK	A4-1	Ra	1
19	OE	C3-2	M	2	RK	A3-2	Sf	1
20	OE	C4-2	M	2	RK	A4-2	Sf	1

Lettertypes:
HT = higher text
TD = three-dimensional
BL = block
SH = shaded
OE = Old English
RK = roman small (lower case version)

Word type:
C = concrete words
A = abstract words
The first numeral is the number of letters the word consists of; the second digit designates the degree of difficulty.

Tasks:
M = same/different
N = naming
Sf = spell forwards
Sb = spell backwards
Ra = request letter position
Rb = request presence of letter in a word

Number of words = the number of words that appear, per presentation, on the screen.

FIGURE 20. An overview of a treatment across 20 sessions in which hemisphere-specific stimulation by means of words is applied via the visual half-fields.

9. The trainer will now retrieve the next set of words from the computer's memory.
10. The trainer presses the key for the first word of the new set.

7.5. Concluding Remarks

There are certain points in the above-described treatment that require further elaboration. The reader will have noticed that for L-dyslexics, *words* are presented in the left visual field and are *concrete* in meaning; also, *complex lettertypes* are used. Concrete words refer to objects and shapes, which are considered to rely more heavily on right hemispheric processing than do abstract words. Similarly, perceptually complex lettertypes are believed to appeal to right hemispheric activity. *Word pairs,* which are to be evaluated as identical or not, are presented with the same objective in mind. This type of evaluation *can* occur on the basis of *word form,* and therefore, the right hemisphere could play a dominating role in the execution of this task. And finally, L-dyslexics hear their own voice (as well as that of the trainer) in the left ear, so that the spoken words are, insofar as is possible, projected to the right hemisphere, as are the words presented visually in the left field. Thus one can ensure that the choice of words (concrete meaning and complex lettertypes) as well as the manner of presentation (left visual and auditory) reflect the goal of activating primarily the right hemisphere.

In contrast, in the case of P-dyslexics, the goal is to prevent any special appeal to right hemispheric activity: Instead of concrete words, abstract words, printed in a perceptually simple print, are flashed one at a time in the right visual field. By asking questions pertaining to letter sequence and by calling upon speech sound analysis, one can activate primarily the left hemisphere.

One might wonder, at this point, whether the pattern of stimulation is so complex that it would not be possible to ascertain precisely which element within the pattern is primarily responsible for the effects on hemispheric activity and scholastic achievement. This observation is, in principle, correct, but the four alternative treatment methods described in Chapter 5 provide a partial answer. The results of these control treatments suggest that perceptual complexity, when isolated from lateral stimulation, had less of an effect in L-dyslexics than when the two were combined. However, it would still be useful to conduct an experiment in which, for example, the effects of lateral auditory (via left and right ear) and lateral visual (via left and right visual field) stimulation were compared with each other.

The preceding sections elaborate the experimental aspects of a treatment method tested by ourselves. The computer programing of this type of treatment method demands considerable time and expertise, which was contributed by one of our colleagues, Rien Moerland (MA). It has gradually become apparent that the procedure can be simplified; for example, we have already mentioned the control of fixation (see Sec. 7.2). Because the program is still in the formative stage, we have not published the software. Rather, we have developed a new program which includes a simpler fixation-control procedure (following Dr. Morris's suggestion; see Sec. 7.2) and which has options for the presentation of any word in any language and for the presentation of (colored) figures. This program, developed by Rien Moerland, is MS-DOS driven and suitable for IBM System 2 personal computers.*

* Program "HEMSTIM" and English manual will be available in 1990. For information/orders: HEMSTIM, Pedological Institute, Department of Child Neuropsychology, P.O. Box 303, 1115 ZG Duivendrecht, Netherlands.

8

Hemisphere-Specific Stimulation (HSS) via the Hands

8.1. Overview

The right hemisphere (for L-dyslexics) and the left hemisphere (for P-dyslexics) are directly accessible not only via the visual half-fields but also via the touch (tactile) receptors of the hands. The experience that has been gained thus far with tactile HSS has been more varied but somewhat less controlled than that obtained with visual HSS (see Chapter 7).

Tactile stimulation has been used by Buyle and Van Dycke (1982), Damen (1983), Caris and Van den Bossche (1983), Notermans and Van de Rijdt (1984), among others, and by many remedial teachers (see Chap. 5, Sec. 5.5). These studies differ from one another with respect to method. Whereas one study used three-dimensional, capital and lower-case letters made of hard plastic (3 mm thick), others used letters constructed from diverse types of material (foamed plastic, soft sponge, felt, cardboard). Damen even fabricated letterforms out of organic material, such as beans, peas, and grains of rice. Some worked with block letters as well as italics, and in everyone's experience the block letters, especially the capitals, were more easily recognized by the children than were the italics. The dimensions of the letters varied considerably and ranged from 9 (lower-case letters) to 25 mm (capitals). Some of the homemade lettertypes—made of felt, for example—were even larger in size (up to 45 mm).

When using letters and other materials to be presented to the

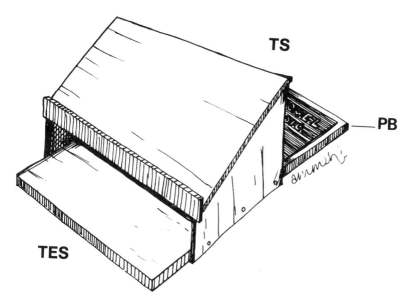

FIGURE 21. A tactile training box, which can be used for hemisphere-specific stimulation via the hands. PB, planning board; TS, trainer's side; TES, trainee's side.

touch, one can employ various kinds of backgrounds on which to place these materials. A *planning board* was frequently used in the studies mentioned above. It is a soft plastic board with grooves in it, on which the materials can be fastened. It comes with separate letters (in various dimensions), which can easily and swiftly be fastened in the grooves, either singly as independent letters or grouped as in words and sentences. These planning boards are fairly expensive, however.

The aim of this technique is to present all of the material to the touch, and out of sight. To attain this goal, a *tactile training box* is used (see Figure 21). The tactile training box that we used has a width of approximately 60 cm, a depth of approximately 55 cm, and a largest and smallest height of 30 and 15 cm, respectively. An opening approximately 10 cm high, over the total width of the tactile training box, appears on the trainee's side; on the trainer's side, the opening is approximately 25 cm high. On the trainee's side of the box, strips of wood have been placed under its floor and at the sides. These strips are slightly thicker than the total thickness of the planning board, including the letters (or other materials) that are fastened onto it. The thick strip of wood has been omitted on the trainer's side of the floor, so that there is an open space between the floor of the training box and the surface on which it has been placed (such as a table, for example); the planning board can be shoved into this open space. One can thus equip the entire planning board with words and shove it under the floor of the box so that only the first row of material is exposed. Once the trainee has worked through the first row of material, the board can subsequently be pulled out to reveal the second row, and so forth. The planning boards that we utilized are 30 cm wide and 40 cm deep. To prevent the child from seeing the board once it is pulled out to the last row, by looking over the top of the box, it is wise to indent the floor of the box, on the trainer's side. The child should be able to sit comfortably behind the tactile training box. Thus, the height of the chair should be such that the elbow of the child's arm, which is put into the tactile training box, can rest on the floor of the box.

8.2. Treatment Procedure

The researchers who gave the tactile HSS treatments made use of a wide variety of tasks, the most important feature of these always being the palpation of letters (usually *not* the letters X, x; Y, y; and Q, q), words, and sentences, with the left hand in the case of the L-dyslexics, and with the right hand in the case of the P-dyslexics. The palpation can be done in various ways, but the preferred method is to use the index and/or middle finger. Usually, the letters/words/sentences were identified first by touch and then were subsequently named aloud. Words and sentences were called out usually after the entire word/sentence had been palpated. We, as well as others (De Kruyk, 1984), wonder whether this approach is beneficial for L-dyslexics: They are inclined to guess anyway, and the treatment method might further encourage this practice. For example, having palpated two words of a sentence, an L-dyslexic might attempt to guess the rest of the sentence. It seems appropriate, therefore, to have the L-dyslexic palpate and name the words in a sentence one by one.

Naming tasks such as that described above can be alternated with other tasks. For example, a letter or figure plate is placed on the slanted side (the "desk" side) of the tactile training box. A palpated letter or word is then compared with, for example, four different words or figures on the plate. Questions that could be posed are: Which word/figure on the plate is equivalent to the word you have just felt? Or, which of the words that you can feel is the same as the word/figure that you see here? For the sake of variety, words/letters were written on the fingertips or palms of the child's hand, or the child was required to write the palpated letter/word, with the hand used for palpation, in the air or on a piece of paper. An alternative approach that would appear to be reasonable but has not been tried as yet (at least not by us) involves the use of letter templates that are specifically adapted to various writing methods. One could let the children write these letters, out of sight, by using the templates. Such templates are available for purchase.

Damen (1983) made use of thematic sessions (30–45 min). If, for example, the theme "money" was used, the sessions would commence with an array of coins which had to be distinguished by means of touch. Subsequently, the names of the coins were to be read (by touch) from the planning board, as were sentences such as "I have lots of money." Damen also deleted letters from words and asked the child to guess at the actual word; this would probably be more appropriate for P-dyslexics than for L-dyslexics (see the caveat on guessing by L-dyslexics, discussed earlier in this section).

It is evident that the level of difficulty of the task should be adapted to the child's abilities. Regardless of the child's abilities, however, the treatment should always commence with the presentation of individual capital letters, followed by lower-case letters, and then simple and more complex groups of letters forming words. The words can be constructed of a combination of various letter-types (perceptually complex words for L-dyslexics). The words can have a concrete meaning (for L-dyslexics) or an abstract meaning (for P-dyslexics). Erroneously read words can be presented once again, and in the case of repeated failure the trainer can name the word him- or herself.

8.3. Concluding Remarks (and a Reservation)

It should be clear by now that HSS via the hands can be designed so that L-dyslexics have all information presented to the fingers of the left hand, and P-dyslexics to those of the right hand. Within this basic framework, many variations on the theme—letter–word palpation and naming—are possible. The choice of a particular variation, however, should be determined largely by the type of dyslexia one is dealing with. An L-dyslexic should palpate letters, words, and sentences with the fingers of the left hand, but as mentioned previously, the lettertype and the material from which the letters are composed, can be varied to enhance the perceptual complexity of the text. The words should refer, insofar as is possible, to concrete (i.e., tangible) things. Tasks in which letters and words have to be compared with one another on the basis of perceptual (physical) characteristics are suitable for L-dyslexics. One may, for the sake of variety, have the child feel and name concrete objects, or palpate words and find which picture/word on the plate corresponds with it. In the latter case, one should take care that the child can reach a decision *only after* the last letter of the word on the planning board has been palpated. An example might clarify this. Suppose that the word "mat" is on the planning board, and the words "man," "mat," "mad," and "map" can be found on the wordplate. The child will be able to reach a decision only when he or she has palpated the "t" of "mat" on the planning board. By means of this procedure, our L-dyslexic will be constrained from guessing. Guessing must be prevented insofar as is possible in the case of L-dyslexics. Thus, one should not present the L-dyslexic with words from which letters have been omitted in order to ask subsequently which word it is.

Tasks, such as that just mentioned, would appear to be more suitable for P-dyslexics. P-dyslexics receive all of their information via the fingers of the right hand. The naming of letters, words, and sentences is appropriate, as are questions regarding the serial (temporal) positions of specific letters in a word or of words in a sentence. One can have the child feel a word—"need" for example—and subsequently ask which one of the following words—"deed," "feed," "need"—called out by the trainer, is equivalent to the palpated word.

For L-dyslexics, words that are to be read by touch should be presented to the fingers of the left hand; for P-dyslexics, to the fingers of the right hand. A number of examples have been provided to illustrate what one can do for the sake of variation. These examples *appear* to be suitable for L- as well as P-dyslexics. We say "appear" because the specific effects of each of these alternative tasks on the right versus the left hemisphere have not been investigated systematically; thus some uncertainty remains. Therefore, we shall have to rely on our professional insight into the nature of the tasks and, on that basis, be confident, at least for the time being, that they will (additionally) activate the right or the left hemisphere. For example, asking for the serial position of the letters in a palpated word is an alternative task that is considered to make an *extra* appeal to the left hemisphere. This assumption is based on data in the literature which make it clear that for most people, the perception of temporal order (of verbal material) is controlled primarily by the left hemisphere. It seems obvious that *exercising* temporal perception (additionally) should activate the left hemisphere, although strictly speaking, it has not been demonstrated conclusively.

9

Hemisphere-Alluding Stimulation (HAS)

9.1. Introduction

In hemisphere-alluding stimulation (HAS), the texts and tasks that are used make a demand on either one of the hemispheres. It should again be apparent that the exercises that one gives to an individual child should be congruent with that dyslexic child's abilities.

In our research (see Chap. 5, Sec. 5.3) we used reading material that was written especially for children with reading disabilities. Because only one session was given per week, books that could be read and finished in two sessions, and short stories, were considered preferable. In light of this time schedule, long stories, which would have required several weeks to finish, might have been demotivating because the child would have to pick up where he or she left off with every new session. Within these confines of length, further selection favored those texts that contained short sentences and, on average, short words. The use and subsequent repetition of difficult words in a text also was considered to be a positive selection criterion.

Whatever text one chooses, the modifications that one makes should be determined by the type of dyslexia one is dealing with (See Secs. 9.2 and 9.3).

Besides texts, one can also give a child linguistic exercises and games. Again the exercises employed should be determined by the type of dyslexia one is treating.

After 20 minutes of reading and 10 minutes of doing exercises, there is usually time, within a treatment session, left over for a game.

9.2. HAS for L-Dyslexics

The *texts* one uses should accentuate perceptual aspects as much as possible and suppress the tendency toward reading in a rushed or hurried fashion. To achieve this goal, one can modify the typography of the text. In our investigation (see Chap. 5, Sec. 5.3), we attained satisfactory results by printing capital and small-cap letters of varying dimensions within a single word. We did this by using the standard lettersets available on the Epson MX-80 F/T matrix printer. Thus, by printing the books one wishes to use in this fashion with the help of a microcomputer and printer, one can achieve an effect like that shown in Figure 22 (the reader is referred also to Figure 7). There are no objections to supplementing the text with illustrations (with the help of a computer, for example). The revised texts should be perceptually complex but, at the same time, still be legible. For children with minimal reading ability, the texts should appear less complex (i.e., one type of capital letter and only one type of small-cap letter with a 1:1 ratio, for example) than those used for children with more advanced reading capabilities (i.e., several types of capital and small-cap letters with a 1:1 ratio, for example). Of course, one should prepare the child somewhat in advance, by saying, "Here is a story that looks rather funny because the capital letters and small letters are all mixed up. If you look carefully, however, you will be able to read it. Start reading." If the child makes an error, one can say, "Try once again to look closely at what it says, and read it once again." One should give the child enough time. If the child is unable to work it out on his or her own, the trainer should read the word first and then ask the child to read the word.

After the texts have been read, the child is given *exercises,* which should be chosen (or modified, if necessary) to ensure that perceptual aspects prevail. In order to make a good choice, one should actually refer to task analyses. If these are lacking, however, one will have to choose on the basis of experience and com-

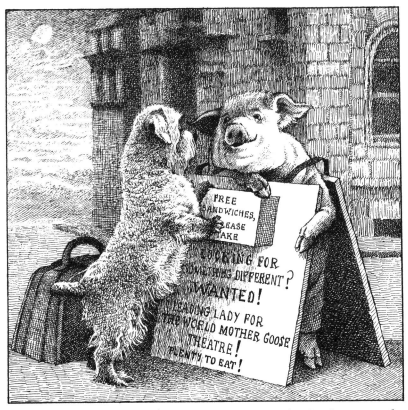

Jennie took everything and went out into the world. On the corner she met a small pig wearing large sandwich boards. He smiled and pointed to a box attached to the front board on which was printed: Free sandwiches, please Take. Jennie chose a tuna on rye and gobbled it as she read the advertisement on the board.

FIGURE 22. Hemisphere-alluding stimulation by means of perceptually complex texts, can be used in dyslexics of the L type. (After M. Sendak, *Higgelty Piggelty Pop, or There Must Be More to Life*, New York: Harper & Row, 1967.)

mon sense. If possible, one should attempt to verify one's choice by checking the literature for tasks of similar perceptual complexity. In our investigation, we used a variety of tasks, several of which are shown in Figure 23. Obviously the level of difficulty of the exercises should be adapted to the child's abilities.

There are CAPITAL LETTERS
and small letters.
Make a word out of the capital letters.
Do the same for the small letters.

| PcLAYhGiROUldND | _____ _____ |
| sLEtMOrNAaDEw | _____ _____ |

Can you read this?

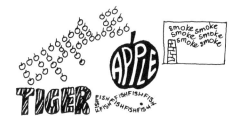

Find the word:
Arrange the bars in the following order: from big to small.
Which word can now be found?

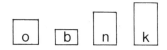

_____

Each box contains five capital letters.
Give each letter a different color.

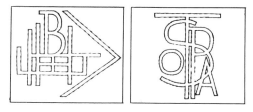

FIGURE 23. Examples of exercises for L-dyslexics. (After Van der Geest & Swuste, 1975; ref. 162.)

9.3. HAS for P-Dyslexics

The reading texts to be given to P-dyslexics should be printed in black ink on white paper and in a typeface that is familiar to the child; any possible perceptual challenge must be avoided. It is best to avoid the use of illustrations. In our investigation (see Chap. 5, Sec. 5.3), a number of words were deleted from the texts (Fig. 24), and the child was requested to fill in the words him- or herself. This was done in an attempt to increase *semantic* skills. With this same goal in mind, questions were posed, during reading, about the meaning of certain words; likewise, after completion of a story, questions about the content of the story were raised.

Before starting to read, the child was told the following: "Here is a story which you may read in a moment. While you are reading, I will occasionally ask you a question. Once in awhile you will notice that there is a word missing from the text, which you must fill in yourself. You may start reading." When reading occurred in a spelling-like or stammering fashion, the trainer would say, "So, what does it say . . . ?" If the child did not know, the trainer would say the word for the child. If a substantive (true) error was made, the trainer would say, "That is incorrect. What do you think

LINES AND SQUARES

Whenever I walk in a London street,
I'm ever so careful to watch my [＿＿＿＿＿];
    And I keep in the squares,
    And the masses of bears,
Who wait at the corners all ready to eat
The sillies who tread on the lines of the street
    Go back to their lairs,
    And I say to them, "Bears,
Just look how I'm [＿＿＿＿＿] in all of the squares!"

FIGURE 24. Hemisphere-alluding stimulation, by means of texts from which words have been deleted, can be used in dyslexics of the P type. (After A. A. Milne, *The World of Christopher Robin.* New York: American Book-Stratford Press, 1958.)

Making words that rhyme:

```
dip    -  . . . . . .  -  . . . . . .  -
fly    -  . . . . . .  -  . . . . . .  -
see    -  . . . . . .  -  . . . . . .  -
win    -  . . . . . .  -  . . . . . .  -
```

One of the words does not rhyme:

```
tin      fan      fin      sin        . . . . . . .

full     pull     ball     bull       . . . . . . .
```

The words that make up the sentences have been placed in the wrong order.
Put them back in the right place:

Jack, Jill and on going are
vacation

We by together traveling are
train

They for have looking days
forward been this to

One of the words does not belong in the list:

```
cow   -  snake -  mouse . . . . . . . . . . . . . . . . . . . .
pencil-  pen   -  brush . . . . . . . . . . . . . . . . . . . .
uncle -  neighbor-  aunt . . . . . . . . . . . . . . . .
```

FIGURE 25. Examples of exercises for P-dyslexics. (After Van der
Geest & Swuste, 1975; ref. 162.)

it says? Read it once again." The trainer would read the word if
the child could not give the correct answer, and then had the child
read it again, as well. When a mistake is made, the trainer should
not linger over it for too long. In summary, the assignments should
be such that fluent reading is encouraged through the use of semantic and symbolic text characteristics.

The *exercises* are aimed at increasing the P-dyslexic's phonetic
skills. Rhyming exercises, among others, seem quite suitable for
this purpose. Figure 25 gives some examples of possible exercises
that can be used. One can see, that the exercises are aimed not

only toward phonetic, but also toward semantic and syntactic analyses.

We had the children read for approximately 20 minutes, and then do exercises for approximately 10 minutes. Once again, we should emphasize that all tasks must be adapted to the child's level of ability.

10

Bibliography

10.1. Introduction

We hope that at this point the reader has gained some insight into the neuropsychological methods that can be used in the treatment of certain types of dyslexia. We anticipate that the interested clinician will be able to apply these techniques solely on the basis of the information provided here. Some readers may want to delve further into the subject matter, and for this reason we have provided a comprehensive listing of scientific publications on which this book is based.

These publications include theoretical discussions as well as research reports. Most of them have been written in the English language, and some are rather technical. We hope that the reader will examine and ponder these sources, because only then will the strengths, weaknesses, gaps, and limitations of the model of dyslexia presented in this book, as well as of the treatment methods derived from this model, become apparent.

The list of publications which follows is classified into two major groups: General Sources (subdivided into Published Research, Theses and Unpublished Reports, Evaluations of Therapeutic Research); and Sources Relating to Specific Chapters (grouped by chapter and section), in order to make them more accessible to the reader. Obviously, this distinction is not absolute and is subjective to some extent. Different chapters often make reference to the same publication; therefore, reference numbers are provided, to which the reader is referred to obtain the original, complete citation. It may not come as a surprise to the reader that a large proportion of the publications listed were written by this author.

10.2. General Sources

Published Research

1. Bakker, D. J., Moerland, R., & Goekoop-Hoefkens, M. (1981). Effects of hemisphere-specific stimulation on the reading performance of dyslexic boys: A pilot study. *Journal of Clinical Neuropsychology, 3*, 155–159.
2. Bakker, D. J., & Vinke, J. (1985). Effects of hemisphere-specific stimulation on brain activity and reading in dyslexics. *Journal of Clinical and Experimental Neuropsychology, 7*, 505–525.
3. Bouma, A., Bakker, D. J., & Gardien, C. J. (1988). Hemisphere-specific stimulation through tactile modality in dyslexics. *Journal of Clinical and Experimental Neuropsychology, 10*, 323.
4. Spyer, G., De Jong, A., & Bakker, D. J. (1987). Piracetam and piracetam plus hemisphere-specific stimulation: Effects on the reading performance of two subtyped dyslexic boys. *Journal of Clinical and Experimental Neuropsychology, 9*, 275–276.

Theses and Unpublished Reports

5. Buyle, V., & Van Dycke, V. (1982). Exploratief onderzoek naar de mogelijke therapeutische effecten van haptische laterale stimulering bij de behandeling van linguale leesgestoorde kinderen. *Thesis.* Genth: Higher Institute for Paramedical Professions.
6. Caris, J., & Van den Bossche, N. (1983). Lezen als breinbreker. *Thesis.* Genth Glut: Higher Institute for Paramedical Professions.
7. Damen, H. (1983). Een trainingsprogramma voor dyslectici. *Thesis.* Amsterdam: Free University.
8. De Kruyk, C. (1984). Drie neuropsychologische trainingen van leesgestoorde LOM-kinderen. *Thesis.* Amsterdam: Free University.
9. Gardien, C. J., Bakker, D. J., & Bouma, A. (1988). Behandeling van dyslectische kinderen: Een veldonderzoek. *Unpublished report.* Amsterdam: Free University.
10. Grace, G. (1987). Brief results of pilot study. *Unpublished report.* Victoria, B.C., Canada: University of Victoria.
11. Notermans, A., & Van de Rijdt, J. (1984). Onderzoek naar de behandelingseffecten van hemisfeer-specifieke training op het leesgedrag en de oogbewegingen van kinderen met leesproblemen. *Thesis.* Tilburg: Catholic University.
12. Reitsma, E. (1985). De differentiële effecten van hemisfeer-specifieke stimulering op de ontwikkeling van leesvaardigheid bij dyslectische kinderen. *Thesis.* Amsterdam: Free University.
13. Romein, C. M. H. (1987). Verandering in leesfoutenpatroon van L- en P-type dyslectici als gevolg van hemisfeer-specifieke training. *Thesis.* Amsterdam: Free University.

14. Spyer, G. (1986). Piracetam en hemisfeer-specifieke stimulering bij een L- en een P-type dyslecticus. *Thesis.* Amsterdam: Free University.

15. Ter Voort, K. (1983). Hemisfeer-specifieke training bij drie lees-zwakke meisjes. *Thesis.* Amsterdam: Free University.

Evaluations of Therapeutic Research

16. Aelbrecht, D. (1987). Het balansmodel van Bakker. *Dissertation.* Louvain: Catholic University.

17. Bakker, D. J. (1982). Brain lateralization and reading disabilities. *Mental Retardation Bulletin, 10,* 38–42.

18. Bakker, D. J. (1982). Zwei Typen von Legasthenikern. *Zeitschrift des Bundesverbandes Legasthenie,* LRS, *4,* 5–9.

19. Bakker, D. J. (1984). The brain as a dependent variable. *Journal of Clinical Neuropsychology, 6,* 1–16.

20. Bakker, D. J. (1986). Scholastic effects of hemisphere-specific stimulation in subtyped dyslexics. In I. Flehmig & L. Stern (Eds.), *Child Development and learning behaviour* (pp. 355–359). New York: Fisher Verlag.

21. Bakker, D. J. (1987). Leerstoornissen: Een hoofdstuk uit de neuro-psychologie van het kind. In J. F. Orlebeke, P. J. D. Drenth, R. H. C. Janssen, & C. Sanders (Eds.), *Compendium van de psychologie* (Vol. 9, pp. 109–138). Muiderberg: Dick Coutinho.

22. Bakker, D. J. (1987). Neuropsychological development and remediation of subtyped reading and spelling disorders. *Journal of Clinical and Experimental Neuropsychology, 9,* 256.

23. Bakker, D. J. (1988). Invoking precursors of deficient reading. In R. L. Masland & M. W. Masland (Eds.), *Preschool prevention of reading failure* (pp. 177–184). Parkton, MD: York Press.

24. Bakker, D. J. (1989). Boosting the (dyslexic) brain. In D. J. Bakker & H. Van der Vlugt (Eds.), *Learning disabilities, Vol. 1: Neuropsychological correlates and treatment* (pp. 173–181). Lisse, the Netherlands: Swets & Zeitlinger.

25. Bakker, D. J. (in press). Alleviation of dyslexia by stimulation of the brain. In G. Th. Pavlidis (Ed.), *Dyslexia: Neuropsychological and learning perspectives.* New York: Wiley.

26. Bakker, D. J., & Heiner, J. (1985). Neuropsychologische mogelijk-heden voor dyslexie-behandeling. In A. van der Leij & L. M. Stevens (Eds.), *Dyslexie 1985* (pp. 195–203). Lisse, the Netherlands: Swets & Zeitlinger.

27. Bakker, D. J., & Licht, R. (1986). Learning to read: Changing horses in midstream. In G. Th. Pavilidis & D. F. Fisher (Eds.), *Dyslexia: Its neuropsychology and treatment* (pp. 87–95). New York: Wiley.

28. Bakker, D. J., Van Leeuwen, H. M. P., & Spyer, G. (1987). Neuro-psychological aspects of dyslexia. In D. J. Bakker, C. Wilsher, H. Debruyne, & N. Bertin (Eds.), *Developmental dyslexia and learning disorders* (pp. 30–39). Basel: Karger.

29. Benton, A. L. (1982). Child neuropsychology: Retrospect and pros-

pect. In J. de Wit & A. L. Benton (Eds.), *Perspectives in child study* (pp. 41–61). Lisse, the Netherlands: Swets & Zeitlinger.

30. Fletcher, J. M. (1985). External validation of learning disability typologies. In B. P. Rourke (Ed.), *Neuropsychology of learning disabilities* (pp. 187–211). New York: Guilford Press.

31. Larsen, S. (1982). To former for laeseretardering. *Skolepsykologi, 19,* 129–144.

32. Larsen, S., & Parlenvi, P. (1982). *Barns liv och läsning.* Malmö: Liber-Förlag.

33. Leong, C. K. (1987). *Children with specific reading disabilities.* Lisse, the Netherlands: Swet & Zeitlinger.

34. Morris, R. (1989). Treatment of learning disabilities from a neuropsychological framework. In D. J. Bakker & H. van der Vlugt (Eds.), *Learning disabilities, Vol. 1: Neuropsychological correlates and treatment* (pp. 183–190). Lisse, the Netherlands: Swets & Zeitlinger.

35. Rourke, B. P., Bakker, D. J., Fisk, J. L., & Strang, J. D. (1985). *Child neuropsychology.* New York: Guilford Press.

Sources Relating to Specific Chapters

Chapter 1.1

36. Atrens, D., & Curthoys, I. (1982). *The neurosciences and behaviour.* Sydney: Academic Press.

37. Changeux, J. P. (1985). *Neuronal man: The biology of mind.* New York: Oxford University Press.

38. House, E. L., Pansky, B., & Siegel, A. (1979). *A systematic approach to neuroscience.* New York: McGraw-Hill.

39. Rourke, B. P., Bakker, D. J., Fisk, J. L., & Strang, J. D. (1985). See no. 35.

40. Spreen, O., Tupper, D., Risser, A., Tuokko, H., & Edgell, D. (1984). *Human developmental neuropsychology.* New York: Oxford University Press.

Chapters 1.2 & 1.3

41. Bakker, D. J. (1967). Left–right differences in auditory perception of verbal and non-verbal material by children. *Quarterly Journal of Experimental Psychology, 19,* 334–337.

42. Bakker, D. J. (1968). Ear-asymmetry with monaural stimulation. *Psychonomic Science, 12,* 62.

43. Bakker, D. J. (1979). Ear-asymmetry with monaural stimulation: Relations to lateral dominance and lateral awareness. *Neuropsychologia, 8,* 103–117.

44. Bakker, D. J., & Kappers, E. J. (1988). Dichotic listening and read-

ing (dis)ability. In K. Hugdahl (Ed.), *Handbook of dichotic listening: Theory, methods and research* (pp. 513–526). New York: Wiley.

45. Bakker, D. J., Licht, R., Kok, A., & Bouma, A. (1980). Cortical responses to word reading by right- and left-eared normal and reading-disturbed children. *Journal of Clinical Neuropsychology, 2,* 1–12.

46. Bakker, D. J., Van der Vlugt, H., & Claushuis, M. (1978). The reliability of dichotic ear asymmetry in normal children. *Neuropsychologia, 16,* 753–757.

47. Corballis, M. C., & Beale, I. L. (1976). *The psychology of left and right.* Hillsdale, NJ: Lawrence Erlbaum.

48. Eling, P. (1983). Studies on laterality. *Dissertation.* Nijmegen: Catholic University.

49. Rourke, B. P., Bakker, D. J., Fisk, J. L., & Strang, J. D. (1985). See no. 35.

50. Van der Vlugt, H. (1979). *Lateralisatie van hersenfunkties.* Lisse, the Netherlands: Swets & Zeitlinger.

51. Van der Vlugt, H. (1979). Een goed stel hersenen, wat is dat eigenlijk? In K. Boer & M. Chamalaun (Eds.), *Breinverkenningen* (pp. 250–265). Assen: Van Gorcum.

52. Van de Vijver, F. R., Kok, A., Bakker, D. J., & Bouma, A. (1984). Lateralization of ERP components during verbal dichotic information processing. *Psychophysiology, 21,* 123–134.

Chapter 2.1

53. Downing, J., & Leong, C. K. (1982). *Psychology of reading.* New York: Macmillan.

54. Gibson, E. J., & Levin, H. (1975). *The psychology of reading.* Cambridge, MA: MIT Press.

55. Leong, C. K. (1987). See no. 33.

Chapter 2.2

56. Bakker, D. J. (1973). Hemispheric specialization and stages in the learning to read process. *Bulletin of the Orton Society, 23,* 15–27.

57. Bakker, D. J. (1979). Perceptual asymmetries and reading proficiency. In M. Bortner (Ed.), *Cognitive growth and development* (pp. 134–152). New York: Brunner/Mazel.

58. Bakker, D. J. (1981). A set of brains for learning to read. In K. C. Diller (Ed.). *Individual differences and universals in language learning aptitude* (pp. 65–71). Rowley, MA: Newbury House.

59. Bakker, D. J., & Kappers, E. J. (1988). See no. 44.

60. Bakker, D. J., & Moerland, R. (1981). Are there brain-tied sex differences in reading? In A. Ansara, N. Geschwind, M. Albert, N. Gartell, & A. Galaburda (Eds.), *Sex differences in dyslexia* (pp. 109–117). Towson: Orton Dyslexia Society.

61. Bakker, D. J., Smink, T., & Reitsma, P. (1973). Ear dominance and reading ability. *Cortex, 9,* 301–312.

62. Bakker, D. J., Teunissen, J., & Bosch, J. D. (1976). Development of laterality reading patterns. In R. M. Knights & D. J. Bakker (Eds.), *The neuropsychology of learning disorders: Theoretical approaches* (pp. 207–220). Baltimore: University Park Press.

63. Goldberg, E., & Costa, L. (1981). Hemisphere differences in the acquisition and use of descriptive systems. *Brain and Language, 14,* 144–173.

64. Kappers, E. J. (1986). Structureringstendentie, hemisfeerspecialisatie en leren lezen. *Dissertation.* Utrecht: State University.

65. Sadick, T. L., & Ginsburg, B. E. (1978). The development of the lateral functions and reading ability. *Cortex, 14,* 3–11.

Chapter 2.3

66. Donchin, E., & McCarthy, M. S. (1979). Event-related brain potentials in the study of cognitive processes. In C. L. Ludlow & M. E. Doran-Quine (Eds.), *The neurological bases of language disorders in children* (pp. 109–128). Bethesda: NIH Publication No. 79-440.

67. Licht, R. (1988). Event-related potential asymmetries and word reading in children. *Dissertation.* Amsterdam: Free University.

Chapter 2.4

68. Bakker, D. J. & Licht, R. (1986). See no. 27.

69. Carmon, A., Nachson, I., & Starinsky, R. (1976). Developmental aspects of visual hemifield differences in perception of verbal material. *Brain and Language, 3,* 463–469.

70. Licht, R. (1988). See no. 67.

71. Licht, R. (1989). Reading disability subtypes: Cognitive and electrophysiological differences. In D. J. Bakker & H. Van der Vlugt (Eds.), *Learning disabilities, Vol. 1: Neuropsychological correlates and treatment* (pp. 81–103). Lisse, the Netherlands: Swets & Zeitlinger.

72. Licht, R., Bakker, D. J., Kok, A., & Bouma, A. (1988). The development of lateral event-related potentials (ERPs) related to word naming: A 4 year longitudinal study. *Neuropsychologia, 26,* 327–340.

73. Licht, R., Kok, A., Bakker, D. J., & Bouma, A. (1986). Hemispheric distribution of ERP components and word naming in preschool children. *Brain and Language, 27,* 101–116.

74. Silverberg, R., Gordon, H. W., Pollack, S., & Bentin, S. (1980). Shift in visual field preference for Hebrew words in native speakers learning to read. *Brain and Language, 11,* 99–105.

Chapter 3.1

75. Bakker, D. J. (1979). Hemispheric differences and reading strategies: Two dyslexias? *Bulletin of the Orton Society, 29,* 84–100.

76. Bakker, D. J. (1981). Cerebral lateralization and reading proficiency. In Y. Lebrun & O. Zangwill (Eds.), *Lateralization of language in the child* (pp. 138–144). Lisse, the Netherlands: Swets & Zeitlinger.

77. Bakker, D. J. (1982). Hemisphere-specific dyslexia models. In R. N. Malatesha & L. C. Hartlage (Eds.), *Neuropsychology and cognition* (Vol. 1, pp. 113–127). Alphen a/d Rijn: Sijthoff & Noordhoff.

78. Bakker, D. J. (1982). Comment: Riding the right hemisphere. In J. de Wit & A. L. Benton (Eds.), *Perspectives in child study* (pp. 73–75). Lisse, the Netherlands: Swets & Zeitlinger.

79. Bakker, D. J. (1982). Cognitive deficits and cerebral asymmetry. *Journal of Research and Development in Education, 15,* 48–54.

80. Bakker, D. J. (1983). Hemispheric specialization and specific reading retardation. In M. Rutter (Ed.), *Developmental neuropsychiatry* (pp. 498–506). New York: Guilford Press.

81. Bakker, D. J. (1987). See no. 21.

82. Bakker, D. J., & Licht, R. (1986). See no. 27.

83. Gaddes, W. H. (1985). *Learning disabilities and brain function.* New York: Springer.

84. Goldberg, E., & Costa, L. (1981). See no. 63.

85. Hynd, G., & Cohen, M. (1983). *Dyslexia.* New York: Grune & Stratton.

86. Rourke, B. P. (1982). Central processing deficiencies in children: Towards a developmental neuropsychological model. *Journal of Clinical Neuropsychology, 4,* 1–18.

87. Rourke, B. P., Bakker, D. J., Fisk, J. L., & Strang, J. D. (1985). See no. 35.

Chapter 3.2

88. Bakker, D. J. (1982). See no. 18.

89. Bakker, D. J. (1973). See no. 56.

90. Bakker, D. J. (1981). See no. 58.

91. Bakker, D. J., Moerland, R., & Goekoop-Hoefkens, M. (1981). See no. 1.

92. Bakker, D. J., Teunissen, J., & Bosch, J. D. (1976). See no. 62.

93. Bakker, D. J., & Vinke, J. (1985). See no. 2.

94. Diller, L., Ben-Yishay, Y., Gerstman, L. J., Goodkin, R., Gordon, W., & Weinberg, J. (1974). *Studies in cognition and rehabilitation in hemiplegia.* New York: New York University Medical Center.

Chapter 3.3

95. Bakker, D. J. (1986). Electrophysiological validation of L- and P-type dyslexia. *Journal of Clinical and Experimental Neuropsychology, 8,* 133.

96. Bakker, D. J., & Licht, R. (1986). See no. 27.

97. Bakker, D. J., Van Leeuwen, H. M. P., & Spyer, G. (1987). See no. 28.

98. Bakker, D. J., Licht, R., Kok, A., & Bouma, A. (1980). See no. 45.

99. Bakker, D. J., & Vinke, J. (1985). See no. 2.

100. Donders, J., & Van der Vlugt, H. (1984). Eye-movement patterns in disabled readers at two age levels: A test of Bakker's balance model. *Journal of Clinical Neuropsychology, 6,* 241–256.

101. Fletcher, J. M. (1985). See no. 30.

102. Lintstra, A. (1983). Event-related potentials and the assessment of brain function: Een verkennend onderzoek naar de samenhang tussen verdubbeling van de vroege negatieve component en dyslexie in het kader van het balansmodel van D. J. Bakker. *Thesis.* Amsterdam: Free University.

103. Notermans, A., & Van de Rijdt, J. (1984). See no. 11.

104. Reitsma, E. (1985). See no. 12.

105. Van Strien, J. W., Bakker, D. J., Bouma, A., & Koops, W. (1988). Familial antecedents of P- an L-type dyslexia. *Journal of Clinical and Experimental Neuropsychology, 10,* 323.

Chapter 3.4

106. Van der Meer, D. J. (1987). Hinken op twee gedachten: Een nadere differentiatie van het P- en L-type. *Thesis.* Amsterdam: Free University.

Chapters 4.1 & 4.2

107. Bakker, D. J. (1986). See no. 20.

108. Bakker, D. J. (1989). See no. 24.

109. Bakker, D. J. (in press). See no. 25.

110. Bakker, D. J., Moerland, R., & Goekoop-Hoefkens, M. (1981). See no. 1.

111. Bakker, D. J., & Vinke, J. (1985). See no. 2.

112. Van den Honert, D. (1977). A neuropsychological technique for training dyslexics. *Journal of Learning Disabilities, 10,* 21–27.

Chapter 4.3

113. Bakker, D. J. (1983). Het hoofd geschoold. In J. de Wit, H. Bolle, & J. M. van Meel (Eds.), *Psychologen over het kind* (Vol. 7, pp. 1–10). Lisse, the Netherlands: Swets & Zeitlinger.

114. Bakker, D. J. (1984). See no. 19.

115. Bakker, D. J. (1987). Hersenen met ervaring. In F. Dijs (Ed.), *Natuurwetenschap in het theater* (pp. 108–125). Amsterdam: Van Gennep.

116. Bakker, D. J. (1987). De mens: Een hoofd vol ervaring. In M. A. Maurice (Ed.), *De mens: Brein onder invloed* (pp. 20–39). Kampen, the Netherlands: Kok.

117. Bakker, D. J. (1989). See no. 24.

118. Diamond, M. C. (1984). A love affair with the brain. *Psychology Today,* November, 62–73.

119. Frostig, M., & Maslow, T. (1979). Neuropsychological contributions to education. *Journal of Learning Disabilities, 12,* 40–54.

120. Greenough, W. T., & Juraska, J. M. (1979). Experience-induced changes in brain fine structure: Their behavioral implications. In M. E. Hahn, C. Jensen, & B. C. Dudek (Eds.), *Development and evolution of brain size* (pp. 295–320). New York: Academic Press.

121. Rosenzweig, M. R., Bennett. E. L., & Diamond. M. C. (1972). Brain changes in response to experience. *Scientific American, 226.* 22–30.

122. Rourke, B. P., Bakker, D. J., Fisk, J. L., & Strang, J. D. (1985). See no. 35.

123. Touwen, B. C. L. (1981). Recovery of neurologically deviant infants. In M. W. van Hof & G. Mohr (Eds.). *Functional recovery from brain damage* (pp. 77–94). Amsterdam: Elsevier/North-Holland.

124. Walsh, R. N. (1981). *Towards an ecology of the brain.* Lancaster, U.K.: M.T.P. Press.

125. Walsh, R. N., & Greenough, W. T. (Eds.). (1976). *Environments as therapy for brain dysfunction.* New York: Plenum.

Chapter 5.1

126. Huck, S. W., Cormier, W. H., & Bounds, W. G. (1974). *Reading statistics and research.* New York: Harper & Row.

127. Morris, R. (1989). See no. 34.

Chapters 5.2–5.6

128. Bakker, D. J., Moerland, R., & Goekoop-Hoefkens, M. (1981). See no. 1.

129. Bakker, D. J., Van Leeuwen, H. M. P., & Spyer, G. (1987). See no. 28.

130. Bakker, D. J., & Vinke, J. (1985). See no. 2.

131. Bakker, D. J., Wilsher, C., Debruyne, H., & Bertin, N. (Eds.). (1987). *Developmental dyslexia and learning disorders.* Basel: Karger.

132. Bouma, A., Bakker, D. J., & Gardien, C. J. (1988). See no. 3.

133. Buyle, V., & Van Dycke, V. (1982). See no. 5.

134. Caris, J., & Van den Bossche, N. (1983). See no. 6.

135. Damen, H. (1983). See no. 7.

136. De Kruyk, C. (1984). See no. 8.

137. Donders, J., & Van der Vlugt, H. (1984). See no. 100.

138. Gardien, C. J., Bakker, D. J., & Bouma. A. (1988). See no. 9.

139. Grace, G. See no. 10.

140. Notermans, A., & Van de Rijdt, J. (1984). See no. 11.

141. Spaninks, H., & Van der Vlugt, H. (1981). Analyses of eye-movement recordings. *Journal of Clinical Neuropsychology, 3,* 331–343.

142. Ter Voort, K. (1983). See no. 15.

Chapters 6.1 & 6.2

143. Bradley, L., & Bryant, P. (1985). *Rhyme and reason in reading and spelling*. Ann Arbor: University of Michigan Press.
144. Licht, R. (1988). See no. 67.
145. Morris, R. (1989). See no. 34.
146. Notermans, A., & Van de Rijdt, J. (1984). See no. 11.
147. Rourke, B. P. (Ed.). (1985). *Neuropsychology of learning disabilities*. New York: Guilford Press.
148. Reitsma, E. (1985). See no. 12.
149. Rutledge, L. T. Synaptogenesis: Effects of synaptic use. In M. R. Rosenzweig & E. L. Bennett (Eds.), *Neural mechanism of learning and memory*, (pp. 329-339). Cambridge, MA: MIT Press.
150. *Theses*. See nos. 7, 11, 12, & 15.

Chapters 7.1–7.5

151. Bakker, D. J., & Vinke, J. (1985). See no. 2.
152. Van den Berg, R. M., & Te Lintelo, H. G. (1977). *A. V. I.-pakket*. Den Bosch: K. P. C.

Chapters 8.1 & 8.2

153. Bouma, A., Bakker, D. J., & Gardien, C. J. (1988). See no. 3.
154. Buyle, V., & Van Dycke, V. (1982). See no. 5.
155. Caris, J., & Van den Bossche, N. (1983). See no. 6.
156. Damen, H. (1983). See no. 7.
157. De Kruyk, C. (1984). See no. 8.
158. Gardien, C. J., Bakker, D. J., & Bouma, A. (1988). See no. 9.
159. Notermans, A., & an de Rijdt, J. (1984). See no. 11.

Chapters 9.1–9.3

160. Bakker, D. J., & Vinke, J. (1985). See no. 2.
161. In den Kleef, H. M. Th. (1975). *Auditieve training: Curriculum schoolrijpheid 2 A*. Den Bosch: Malmberg.
162. Van der Geest, A. N., & Swuste, W. (1975). *Taalverwerkingsprogramma*. Den Bosch: Malmberg.

Index

Italic *f* following a page number denotes a figure.